Narrative-based Primary Care

A practical guide

John Launer

Senior Lecturer in General Practice and Primary Care
Tavistock Clinic

Foreword by

Professor Trisha Greenhalgh

Radcliffe Medical Press

Radcliffe Medical Press Ltd
18 Marcham Road
Abingdon
Oxon OX14 1AA
United Kingdom

www.radcliffe-oxford.com
The Radcliffe Medical Press electronic catalogue and online ordering facility.
Direct sales to anywhere in the world.

British Library Cataloguing in Publication Data

A catalogue record for this book is available from the British Library.

ISBN 1 85775 539 1

Typeset by Aarontype Ltd, Easton, Bristol
Printed and bound by TJ International Ltd, Padstow, Cornwall

Contents

Foreword

Many years ago, when I was a newly registered GP, I saw Sharyn Prentice, a 15-year-old girl of West Indian origin, in evening surgery. She attended with a friend; both were in school uniform and blowing bubble gum. There was a lot of whispering and giggling between them, and in the end I asked them if they would like to write the problem down. Sharyn's friend scribbled down the single word 'pregnant' on a piece of paper, folded it over tightly and handed it to me without looking up.

The information came as no surprise. Sharyn had been an erratic attender for her contraceptive prescriptions, and her mother had once wearily described her as 'forward'. I asked Sharyn if her mum knew about the pregnancy. 'Yes', she said, looking at her friend and giggling again. I confirmed the diagnosis and examined Sharyn, who did not appear to be more than 9 weeks pregnant.

I knew Sharyn's family fairly well. She was the eldest of nine children who lived in a rambling old house backing on to the railway. I had seen Mrs Prentice for her latest postnatal check only a month ago. I had never met the father, but the younger Prentice siblings were a lively, confident and tough brood, whose appearance en masse in the waiting room struck fear into the hearts of the less-experienced receptionists.

I asked Sharyn if her mum would agree to her having an abortion. 'I'm sure she would', she said. I filled out a form for a dating scan and completed the legally required paperwork for a termination of pregnancy, confirming that, in my opinion, the continuation of the pregnancy would pose considerable hazard to the mental health of the mother. I phoned through and made a provisional appointment for an emergency consultation at the community gynaecology unit. I wrote the details of the appointment on the outside of the envelope and asked Sharyn to tell her mother to contact me if there was a problem.

I didn't see Sharyn for six months, and assumed that the procedure had gone ahead. Then, in another late evening surgery, she attended as an emergency, again with her schoolfriend, saying she couldn't get her ring off and her finger was hurting. To my horror, I noted that Sharyn's hands (and, incidentally, her face, legs and feet too) showed a dramatic degree of oedema. She was now 32 weeks pregnant, and her diastolic blood pressure was 120. She was clearly in an advanced state of pre-eclampsia. I called an ambulance and rushed Sharyn in for specialist care. She had a 1.5 kg baby girl, Lola, by caesarean section the next day.

Over the next two months, Sharyn visited Lola five times a day by bus, taking a gift of expressed breast milk each time. She read her baby endless stories from nursery books and took dozens of pictures with a cheap instamatic camera. When I visited the special care baby unit, the nurses commented that they had rarely seen a more devoted mother. When the infant was finally discharged, she was absorbed into the large, chaotic and supportive Prentice family, and Sharyn returned to school to prepare for her GCSE examinations. When she came to the surgery, she invariably brought tiny Lola in a papoose sling and displayed her proudly to all the staff.

After a few months, I asked her why she had failed to attend for antenatal care. 'Because', she said, 'you told me to go for an abortion.'

'But why didn't you tell me you wanted to keep the baby?', I asked.

'Because you didn't ask. And I don't think I was sure then anyway.'

Sharyn's story (her details have been changed to protect confidentiality) had a happy ending. But Sharyn and her daughter very nearly paid the ultimate price for my attempt to impose a professional, white middle-class narrative on the predicament she so tentatively shared with me. She had come to me with a half-told story, and my own unconscious enthusiasm to pen the next chapter left her own hopes, dreams and fears unexplored.

Sharyn taught me a lot about what it means to be 15, black and pregnant. It didn't mean what I had originally thought it meant. She also taught me what it means to be deprived of choices by well-meaning health professionals; what it means to be part of a big, happy family in which everyone pulls together; and what it means to combine responsible motherhood with the continuing adventures and uncertainties of adolescence.

Like most trainee GPs, I viewed my early consultations in general practice as discrete episodes to be addressed by the biomedical, doctor-driven, problem-solving approach that I had brought from my hospital training. Like most experienced GPs, I have subsequently learnt to accommodate my biomedical knowledge and skills within a more continuous interpretative and therapeutic framework that acknowledges the uniqueness and value of the patient's story and builds towards new instalments of an evolving (and collaborative) narrative. Even now, I am aware that precious few of my consultations fulfil Launer's criteria for a 'good story' – coherence, narrative (aesthetic) appeal and practical value.

I learnt a lot from this book, both about the philosophical basis of the narrative approach and (perhaps more usefully) about simple, practical techniques to use in the consulting room. Sharyn might have been spared many of the complications of her high-risk pregnancy if I had given her the opportunity to consider some questions from the list on page 40 – speculative ('What would happen if …'), ranking ('What is the most/least …') and relational ('What effect would this have on your family …'). I should, of course, have reflected on her story so far, strategised the conversation so that she could develop it further, and empowered her to tell me what she wanted to do.

As Launer says, there is no fast-track route or fail-safe formula for the effective use of narrative in clinical practice. It will take time to develop the necessary skills, and both the trainee and the more experienced practitioner can expect to produce some pretty poor stories along the way. We must remain reflective, curious and humble – and we must recognise the need to share the narratives from our own encounters with a mentor, colleague or peer learning group, both for our own professional development and (in the wider scheme of things) for the purposes of generating new knowledge and new theory.

General practitioners live in exciting times. I am sure this book will quickly find its place on the shelf of key textbooks on the core values and methods of primary healthcare. As Launer rightly claims in Chapter 14, the narrative approach – whose distinguishing feature might be defined as inter-subjectivity – supplements and builds on the range of models of the consultation developed by Byrne and Long, Pendleton, Stott and Davies, Stewart and other names with which the student of academic general practice is already familiar.

John Launer has wisely avoided presenting any of his ideas as the 'last word' on this rapidly expanding subject. There is much theoretical work still to be done to place narrative-based medicine in its appropriate epistemological niche at the intersection of several disciplines including linguistics, sociology, psychology, family therapy, psychoanalysis and biomedicine. There is a huge educational agenda at both undergraduate and postgraduate level – how can different practitioners best learn the techniques of narrative, apply them in practice, demonstrate their competence and improve their performance year on year? And there is a challenging research agenda – how can we refine these narrative techniques and evaluate their acceptability and usefulness in the many different cultures and contexts represented in primary healthcare and beyond? Launer does not seek to provide simple answers to these questions in this book. But those who find themselves grappling with the academic challenges of narrative health research over the next few years will find that the chapters that follow provide a pioneering map of the territory and set the stage for further work.

Professor Trisha Greenhalgh OBE
Professor of Primary Health Care
University College London
April 2002

Preface

We understand ourselves inescapably in narrative.
Charles Taylor (1989)

This is a book about primary care, and about the stories that are told there. In this preface I want to explain how the book came to be written, its purpose and its structure.

One evening 20 years ago, I was with some friends in a north London pub listening to the Crouch End All Stars playing jazz. In a break between numbers, my friends introduced me to the banjo player – a local GP called Hilary Graham. I asked him if he was looking for a trainee. Hilary enquired if I had a driving licence. When I said yes, he agreed to become my GP trainer. Then he climbed back on to the stage to play the next piece. How simple things were in those days!

As well as taking risks, Hilary was an inspired and prescient GP. He was one of the first GPs in Britain to become interested in family therapy (Graham 1991). Occasionally during my trainee year, he would refer a family to Sebastian Kraemer at the Tavistock Clinic. We would both go along with the family. I was impressed by what I saw. When I joined my own practice, I continued to take a few families there too. The Tavistock had one of the few child and family clinics in the NHS that welcomed GPs taking part in this way. Later, Sebastian encouraged me to enrol on the introductory course at the Institute of Family Therapy, where I learned some basic family therapy ideas and techniques to use in the surgery.

It is tempting to present a story as a smooth sweep of progress, but things were not like that. By the late 1980s, I was feeling depressed by my work and in danger of professional burnout. This was partly because of the NHS changes and partly for other reasons. I had also been seriously ill with myocarditis. In 1991, I decided to take a year off. I was uncertain how to spend it. However, through a series of conversations and opportunities I was offered a place on the clinical training in family therapy at the Tavistock. The training transformed my view of my work, and of primary care itself. When I started my sabbatical, I had been unsure if I would return to general practice. When I finished it, I was certain that I wanted to remain a GP and convinced that family therapy and primary care could learn a huge amount from each other.

My tutor at the Tavistock was Caroline Lindsey, a child psychiatrist as well as a family therapist. She became fascinated by primary care. Together, we thought up the notion of using ideas from family therapy – particularly ideas about systems, contexts and narratives – as a way of conceptualising the whole work of primary care. We felt that this could potentially transform the way people worked in that setting. We hoped it could do so not by turning them into amateur family therapists, but by offering a different view of their work: as facilitators of stories. In order to explore this notion, we first carried out some research into the consultation to explore these ideas (Launer 1995). Encouraged by what we found, we set up a postgraduate course for primary care professionals (Launer and Lindsey 1997). Caroline has now become a good friend as well as an inspiring collaborator in the work in all its dimensions: training, research, theory and practice. She first suggested the idea for this book. Everything in it bears the stamp of conversations with her, and of the seven years of teaching that we have done together in developing a narrative approach to primary care.

The book is based on our courses. All the ideas in it have been developed with the people who have come on them: mainly GPs and practice nurses, but also health visitors and community nurses, pharmacists, optometrists and dentists. The aim of the book is not to suggest that such training is the only way that people can become narrative-based practitioners. It is to make the ideas better known, so that people can try them out for themselves in their own work and integrate them into their existing forms of practice if they wish. The book may also be useful for educators wishing to teach similar approaches.

Like the courses, this book offers a particular approach to understanding primary care, to practising it and to teaching it. It addresses some of the crucial questions that people in primary care are asking in the 21st century, such as:

- How do you practise primary care when the authority of medicine and of professionals including doctors can no longer be taken for granted?
- How can you share power with patients, without letting go of evidence and science?
- How do you work alongside colleagues who may have other views, other beliefs and perhaps other professions?
- How can you practise humanely while following a huge agenda of preventive medicine, disease surveillance and keeping to guidelines?
- How can you hold on to optimism about the possibility of change when you see so many people who are intractably distressed?
- How can you manage all of this when time and resources are so short?
- How can you be a care professional and remain a caring person?

Although the book is based on narrative ideas from family therapy, the main focus is on their practical application to ordinary consultations with individuals, working in a seven- or ten-minute time slot. It is also on how these ideas might help practices, partnerships and teams in their wider work, including teaching, supervision and team building. It is an attempt to take the challenges of narrative ideas seriously, while paying proper respect to the realities of primary care. One theme runs through the book: *the main role of primary care is to help people to develop new narratives for themselves.*

This book makes no claim to present the *only* way of using narrative ideas in primary care. A number of other people have now proposed innovative approaches in this setting, using narrative ideas (Borkan *et al.* 2001; Frank 1998; Heath 1998). Nor does the book make any pretence of covering the field of studies concerning people's accounts of their illness experiences: this area is amply and expertly covered in many outstanding books and articles (Kleinman 1988; Frank 1995; Mattingly and Garro 2000; Bury 2001). It is also not about a particular style of 'narrative therapy' currently practised by some eminent family therapists (White and Epston 1990). While drawing on many different sources, including all of those mentioned, it is primarily an attempt to present one particular approach that has been specifically developed for daily practice in primary care.

Some readers may well read the examples of good narrative practice and see a resemblance to other contemporary approaches in primary care such as patient enablement and shared decision making (Howie *et al.* 1997, 2000; Towle and Godolphin 1999; Elwyn *et al.* 1999; Edwards and Elwyn 2001) . They may notice similarities to other fields they know about, like complexity or chaos theory (Plsek and Greenhalgh 2001). They may say, 'I do that anyway' or 'That just demonstrates good primary care'. So much the better. It will not be surprising if narrative-based primary care converges with what many practitioners already do intuitively, or by using ideas from other sources. However, it may still offer readers a new and coherent language for conceptualising, practising and teaching primary care.

The structure of this book, and ways to read it

Following a general introduction, the first part of this book is entitled 'Practice'. It presents a simple, straightforward guide to a narrative-based approach for primary care. It is designed as a practical handbook. The key ideas are highlighted at the beginning of each chapter. There are suggested points to consider and exercises to try. Each chapter in this section ends with an extract from one of the articles or books we use as source material and that we sometimes include as set reading on our courses. Most of the section addresses issues in the consultation, but it also looks at clinical supervision and teamwork. The whole section is intentionally didactic but this is meant as a way of stimulating dialogue, not of promulgating dogma.

The second part of this book, 'Teaching', takes a more educational perspective. It provides some background concerning the nature and development of family therapy, its relationship with primary care and the role of the Tavistock Clinic in the National Health Service. It traces the historical origins of the approach and the development of the training. It also describes our method of teaching in some detail and gives an account of some of the effects of the courses.

The third part of this book, 'Theory', addresses theoretical topics. These include comparisons of a narrative approach with patient-centred medicine and the Balint tradition. The last chapter is entitled 'Towards a narrative-based model for primary care'.

All readers will probably benefit from reading the Introduction first, as it explains what this book is about. However, the book can then be read in many different ways, including the following:

- straight through
- by reading Part Two first (particularly for readers who are educators or who prefer to understand an approach in terms of its historical development)
- by reading Part Three first (particularly for readers who have a thirst for theory).

Some readers may also want to dip in and out of the different sections in order to pursue their own preferred learning trajectory. The chapter headings and the index are designed to make this as easy as possible.

The last chapter is an account of the philosophical approach underlying this book and the Appendix describes the research that first led to our training work. Each of these can be read in its own right at any stage.

Readers may be struck by the unconventional order of the three sections: practice, then teaching, then theory. This is intentional. The main emphasis of the book is on applying narrative ideas at the 'coal face'. However, the section topics are by no means watertight. There are some theoretical ideas in the practice and teaching sections, and vice versa. It is impossible to teach well, or to theorise clearly, except from a basis of sound practice. Equally, it is impossible to practise well without standing back at times to extrapolate some intelligent theory: in other words, to develop a cycle of reflective practice (Schon 1983)

This book has grown out of many conversations. The ideas in it have stimulated dialogue, discussion and creative dissent. It is hoped these will all continue. Questions, comments, objections and reflections will all be very welcome and can be sent direct to the author: jlauner@tavi-port.org.

John Launer
April 2002

References

Borkan J, Reis S and Medalie J (2001) Narratives in family medicine: tales of transformation, points of breakthrough for family physicians. *Fam Sys Health.* **19**: 121–34.

Bury M (2001) Illness narratives: fact or fiction? *Soc Health Illn.* **23**: 263–85.

Edwards A and Elwyn G (eds) (2001) *Evidence Based Patient Choice.* Oxford University Press, Oxford.

Elwyn G, Edwards A and Kinnersley P (1999) Shared decision making: the neglected second half of the consultation. *Br J Gen Pract.* **49**: 477–82.

Frank A (1995) *The Wounded Story Teller: body, illness and ethics.* University of Chicago Press, Chicago.

Frank A (1998) Just listening: narrative and deep illness. *Fam Sys Health.* **16**: 197–212.

Graham H (1991) Family interventions in general practice. *J Fam Ther.* **13**: 225–30.

Heath I (1998) Following the story: continuity of care in general practice. In: T Greenhalgh and B Hurwitz (eds) *Narrative Based Medicine: dialogue and discourse in clinical practice.* BMJ Books, London.

Howie JGR, Heaney DJ and Maxwell M (1997) *Measuring Quality in General Practice: occasional paper 75.* Royal College of General Practitioners, London.

Howie JGR, Heaney DJ, Maxwell M and Walker JJ (2000) Developing a 'consultation quality index' (CQI) for use in general practice. *Fam Pract.* **17**: 455–61.

Kleinman A (1988) *The Illness Narratives: suffering, healing and the human condition.* Basic Books, New York.

Launer J (1995) A social constructionist approach to family medicine. *Fam Sys Med.* **13**: 379–89.

Launer J and Lindsey C (1997) Training for systemic general practice: a new approach from the Tavistock Clinic. *Br J Gen Pract.* **47**: 453–6.

Mattingly C and Garro LC (eds) (2000) *Narrative and the Cultural Construction of Illness and Healing.* University of California Press, California.

Plsek P and Greenhalgh T (2001) The challenge of complexity and health care. *BMJ.* **323**: 625–8.

Schon D (1983) *The Reflective Practitioner: how professionals think in action.* Temple Smith, London.

Taylor C (1989) *Sources of the Self: the making of the modern identity.* Cambridge University Press, Cambridge.

Towle A and Godolphin W (1999) Framework for teaching and learning informed shared decision making. *BMJ.* **319**: 766–71.

White M and Epston D (1990) *Narrative Means to Therapeutic Ends.* Norton, New York.

Acknowledgements

Many of the teachers on the primary care course at the Tavistock Clinic over the past seven years have contributed ideas that appear in these pages. Apart from Caroline Lindsey and myself as organising tutors, the teaching staff has included Jenny Altschuler, Sara Barratt, John Byng-Hall, David Campbell, Barbara Dale, Emilia Dowling, Rita Harris, Sebastian Kraemer and Renos Papadopoulos. Since the GP and Primary Care Unit was established at the Tavistock, Jane Rayner and Lucy Ettinger have been enthusiastic in their secretarial and administrative support and have made all the work of the Unit possible.

It is no mere cliché to say that people coming on Tavistock courses have taught us as much as we have taught them. This too is reflected in every chapter here. Many past participants have helped with this book by providing examples of cases, or by setting down their thoughts in writing, and I am very grateful to them. They include Paquita de Zulueta, Tessa Dresser, George Farrelly, Anat Gaver, Helen Halpern, Rachel Hopkins, Cath Humphrys, David Masters and Sue Whitehead.

At around the same time that we started our courses, a number of GPs, counsellors and others who were interested in the links between family therapy and primary care were also joining up nationally. These people included Hilary Graham, Robert Mayer, Dave Tomson, Jack Czauderna and Venetia Young. Together, we formed the 'Thinking Families Network'. Similar networks have also sprung up abroad, including those led by Pekka Larivaara in Finland, and Anat Gaver and Amnon Toledano in Israel. These networks have been an important source of inspiration and comradeship along the way and have helped to inform this book. So have the psychologists who have done collaborative work with me in primary care, either clinically or through research. I particularly want to acknowledge the contributions of Emilia Dowling, Alan Nance and Amal Treacher.

None of this work would have been possible, or have made any sense, without maintaining a solid base in general practice. For 18 years now, I have had the privilege of working with an exceptional team at the Forest Road Practice in Edmonton, north London, most importantly with Ron Singer, Mary Logan and Sally Jowett. They have gone out of their way to accommodate me as a GP colleague while I acquired a bewildering series of extra identities as family therapist, educator and writer (not to mention husband, rabbinic spouse and father of twins). They have kept me going in good times and bad. So have the hundreds of people who have seen me at Forest Road as general practice patients since 1983. Necessarily anonymous here, they are the principal inspirations for the narrative in these pages.

I am grateful to the current and former editors of journals who have allowed me to adapt material here that has been published elsewhere. Chapters 11 and 12 are based on a series of articles in *Education for General Practice*. Chapter 16 has been adapted from a paper that appeared in the *Journal of Family Therapy* entitled ' "You're the doctor, Doctor!": is social constructionism a useful stance in general practice consultations?'. The appendix reports on research that was previously published in *Families, Systems and Health* with the title: 'A social constructionist approach to family medicine'. Some of the case material has previously been discussed in a lecture on the use of family therapy ideas in community work, published in the Leo Baeck College series *Partners in Leadership* and in *European Judaism*. The chapters relating to patient-centred medicine and the Balint movement are based on a literature review that was funded by the North Central London primary care research network (NoCTeN) and supervised by David Armstrong.

Two people have been unfailingly supportive in promoting the approach to primary care teaching described in this book: they are Jonathan Burton of the London GP Deanery and Andrew Harris of Camden and Islington Health Authority. Trisha Greenhalgh and Brian Hurwitz invited me to contribute to their book *Narrative Based Medicine* and hence sowed an idea for the book. While I have been writing it, several people have been extraordinarily generous with their time and suggestions in order to help me improve it. They have included Ron Singer, Jonathan Burton, Paul Thomas and David Campbell. Paul Sackin kindly commented on the chapter on the Balint approach, although the views expressed there are mine and not his. Gillian Nineham has been as supportive an editor as any author could hope for. Many of the merits of the book may be due to these people. Its failings are mine.

I have had many helpful conversations along the way with one colleague who is neither a family therapist nor in primary care, but intuitively understands both, and much more: Brian Snowdon. His caring and thoughtful influence is pervasive.

As well as being a tactful and challenging reader, my wife Lee Wax has been unwavering in her love and in her encouragement to do the work that lies behind this book, and the book itself. The book is dedicated to her and to our children.

For Lee, for Ruth, for David.

Introduction: narrative and primary care

'To be in a culture is to be bound in a set of connecting stories.'
Jerome Bruner (1990)

'Narrative based medicine is about helping people to tell stories that have to be told if all of us are to remain fully human.'
Arthur Frank (2001)

Key ideas in this introduction

- Narrative ideas can provide a framework for thinking about everything that goes on in primary care, including encounters with patients and encounters between professionals.
- Ideas from family therapy can act as a helpful bridge between narrative thinking from the social sciences and the practical world of primary care.
- Some contemporary thinkers see all knowledge as stories, including science and medicine. People in primary care can make good use of such ideas, while remaining grounded in the world of action and physical facts.

Why narrative?

Story telling is a defining human activity (Bruner 1986). Stories or narratives – the words are interchangeable – unite all cultures, cross all history and arise in all circumstances. Stories in this sense are not fables, lies or fairy tales. They are the way we understand, experience, communicate and indeed create ourselves. They are also the way we try to influence others. They constantly change as people tell them. They consist of the process of telling as well as the end product.

Patients come to primary care because they have problems, but almost invariably they present these problems as a story: '*This happened, and then that happened, and then I felt something . . . I talked to a few people about it . . . Now I want to know what to do.*' In one sense, a story like this is merely the way that people communicate their problems. In another sense, the story itself needs treatment. Patients want to go away with a better story: '*My problem seems less . . . I understand it better . . . now I know what to do.*'

Professionals in primary care tell stories too: '*This is how I see your problem . . . This is what I think you should do about it . . . These tablets will make you feel better.*' Professional stories like these are usually connected to official narratives like biological science and evidence-based medicine (Hunter 1991; Atkinson 1995). Sometimes they provide patients with a better story and sometimes they do not. Either way, we cannot work without narratives. Whatever the task, it is always embedded in a story for the patient and a story for the professional.

Primary care offers multiple opportunities to patients for creating new stories (Cole-Kelly 1992; Launer 2002) The same patient may tell different stories to the receptionist, the practice nurse, the doctor and the cleaner – and will receive many new stories in exchange. None of these stories is definitive, nor are any of them distortions. Each is recreated in a different way, the production of the listener as much as the teller. Primary care offers professionals similar opportunities too, as they create stories about their work, in corridor conversations or team meetings. For both patients and professionals, primary care can be seen as a space for continual narrative reconstruction.

A narrative-based approach sees the search for better stories, and the attempt to provide these, as the basis of all the work that is done in primary care. Narrative ideas offer a conceptual framework for understanding all the different discourses – professional and scientific ones, together with lay or folk accounts of the world – that have to be integrated into everyday work. They can help practitioners to make sense of all the story-telling activities that go on within primary care: not only with patients, but also between colleagues, within teams and throughout the health service. Narrative ideas can also provide practitioners with the skills to help patients and colleagues alike to question, re-evaluate and change their own narratives.

Where the ideas come from

There has been an explosion of ideas about narrative in the past 30 years. This has happened in all kinds of fields: in psychology (Bruner 1986, 1990; Roberts and Holmes 1999), in the humanities (Ricoeur 1984), and in the social sciences (Geertz 1973). In all these subjects, the focus has moved away from observing the content of people's lives to examining the processes of living. These processes are nearly always characterised by speaking and thinking in a flow of words. The world of narrative studies is now vast. People have studied how we construct our memories and our life stories in a similar way to authors writing novels: with time frames, characters and themes, and with elements such as plots and suspense (Mattingly 1998). They have examined how we present ourselves to others in narrative form (Riessman 1990). They have looked at how our stories change as time passes, and how they change as we have conversations with others.

Many ideas about narrative have a 'postmodern' flavour. Postmodernism rejects overarching accounts of reality (Lyotard 1984). It challenges the objectivity of science and medicine. It understands all knowledge as the product of culture: in other words, as stories that will one day cease to have meaning – just as we no longer believe the 'obvious' story that the sun goes round the earth. Postmodernist thinkers reject the idea that exploring reality is like peeling away the layers of an onion, looking for the inner meaning concealed at the centre. Instead, they see it more like a tapestry of language that is continually being woven. This way of looking at language and reality is sometimes called *social constructionism* (Berger and Luckman 1966; Gergen and Davis 1985; Harre 1986). Social constructionists believe that it is language that largely determines reality rather than the other way around.

Until quite recently, there was very little interest in these ideas in the medical world. Phrases like 'narrative studies', 'postmodernism' or 'social constructionism' meant nothing to most practitioners, unless they happened to work in departments of medical sociology or anthropology. That has now changed, and it has changed radically. In the past few years, these ideas have arrived on the medical scene with surprising speed. Partly this has come about because of social and political changes that have knocked doctors and other professions off their pedestals (Smith 2001). Partly it is because of movements like feminism and antiracism that have invited people to look at their own beliefs and behaviour, and how these reflect their own vested interests. Consumerism has also had an effect (Lupton 1997; Coulter 1999). So have patient pressure groups and disability rights activists. All these interest groups have different kinds of stories to offer, and they want to be heard.

As a result, most doctors and health professionals are now aware that not everyone thinks that medicine is objective or politically neutral (Hahn and Gaines 1985; Lock and Gordon 1988; Morris 1998). They are coming to accept that professionals do not have a monopoly on describing people's experiences when they are ill, or on telling them what to do about it. The medical press is now full of articles about narratives, postmodernism and social constructionism, and about how doctors should take these on board (Hodgkin 1996; Mathers and Rowland 1997; Muir Gray 1999; Wilson 2000; Calman 2001). There is now a core text on narrative-based medicine (Greenhalgh and Hurwitz 1998).

It provides an excellent introduction to the many points of intersection between the fields of narrative studies and of medicine. There are the beginnings of a narrative-based medicine movement, committed to restoring humanity, imagination, humility and moral engagement to the medical world (Kirmayer 2001). Its aim is to provide a counterbalance to dominant stories like evidence-based medicine, molecular genetics or pharmaceutical science. In some respects, narrative-based medicine turns conventional medical thinking on its head. Instead of listening to 'the patient's history' to determine the right diagnosis and treatment, it judges these by whether they contribute to an improvement in the patient's story.

Family therapy: a bridge between narrative studies and primary care

Taking a narrative-based approach to primary care is a fairly new idea. However, there is one related clinical field where narrative ideas have already had a great influence – the field of family therapy. There is now quite a long history of links between family therapy and general practice. Many of these have involved looking at how people come to primary care and family therapy with similar problems, and might be helped by the same kinds of treatment (some of these links are described later in this book). However, in the past few years it has become clear that family therapy can offer something more to primary care: an example of how to use narrative ideas when dealing with the whole range of everyday work. In other words, it can give some guidance to working professionals about how to take the ideas off the pages of social science textbooks and into the consulting room.

Family therapists have worked hard to deal with the implications of narrative thinking (Anderson and Goolishian 1988; Hoffman 1990; McNamee and Gergen 1992). They have tried to adapt their approach and their techniques to a world where they can no longer take notions like objectivity and authority for granted. They have had to acknowledge the major effects of racial and other kinds of discrimination in their clients' lives, including gender issues (Goldner 1985; Luepnitz 1988; O'Brian 1990). They have had to take the religious beliefs of their clients into account (Walrond-Skinner 1989; Prest and Keller 1993). At the same time, they have tried to respect families' expectations that they should still have some expertise to offer and that they should remain professional, ethical, competent and serious (Fine and Turner 1991). In response to this challenge, they have moved away from theories that try to explain what people and families *should* be like and how they should behave. Instead, they have taken the view that they need to help people explore a range of new realities (Fruggeri 1992; Cecchin *et al*. 1994). They have largely stopped seeing their work as an opportunity to uncover hidden truths and have started to regard it as a chance to explore stories in collaboration with the patient or client. Most family therapy is now based on the idea of asking creative questions to encourage patients to construct new narratives for themselves.

Applying these ideas in primary care

The attractions of such an approach in primary care are clear. It might offer clinicians a respectable intellectual framework for working in the 21st century – a framework that was no longer rooted in 18th century mind/body dualism (McWhinney 1996). It might provide them with a single consistent way of thinking about all the different levels of their activity, including consultations with patients, clinical supervision, training, management work and political negotiation. It might lead them to question some of the apparently solid certainties of science and of medicine. It could give them a new view of such things as diagnosis and evidence, and sensitise them to folk beliefs about illness (Blumhagen 1980; Heurtin-Roberts 1993).

In addition, a narrative approach could help practitioners to become more aware of their social and political roles. It might encourage them to examine the power relations in their encounters with patients and with team members. It might help them to notice how power can be expressed in the subtleties of language, as well as in more obvious ways, such as rudeness or paternalism. It could enrich their work by drawing their attention to the variety of cultures and beliefs with which they come into contact. It might be helpful because it raises their awareness of gender, ethnicity and social class, and alerts them to the experiences of people living in adverse circumstances, such as refugees. It might also assist them to let go of a constant sense of responsibility for other people's problems and to acquire a greater sense of the possibilities open to their patients.

The attractions of this kind of approach in primary care are obvious, but so are the challenges. Patients come to primary care because they want to meet experts who can offer conventional medical explanations for their problems. A narrative approach must provide a way of asking intelligent questions about medical knowledge without disqualifying that knowledge (Launer 1996a). It should help professionals to let go of rigid certainty about medical facts, but it should not make them so uncertain about everything that they feel unable to do their jobs.

Professionals in primary care are not only paid to listen and speak; they also have to do things. They have to stick needles into people, dispense drugs, carry out minor operations, prevent illness, monitor risk and do a host of other business. Patients expect them to be reasonably good counsellors but they also expect them to be technical experts, dealing with bodies as much as with words. A narrative approach cannot exclude action, nor can it be a licence for ignoring all the other normal tasks of primary care, such as giving advice, educating people and offering reassurance. It needs to fit a world where practitioners are regularly crossing over between different activities, such as helping with a marital problem and carrying out an intimate physical examination on the same person within a few days or even minutes.

There is another obvious challenge too. Most people in primary care have to work under tremendous pressure of time and workload. They face demands from health service managers and politicians, as well as resource shortages. There is no point in trying to import narrative ideas and skills into primary care if these only work in consultations lasting an hour, or when seeing patients at regular intervals of every week or two, or by regularly inviting whole families to attend. Nor will they be helpful if they open up a 'Pandora's box' that people do not have the skills or the resources to cope with. To be useful, a narrative approach needs to be adapted specifically for primary care, with all its limitations. It must help people to use short consultations more efficiently rather than putting them under even greater pressure. It must help to combat work stress and burnout instead of turning the screw even further.

The biggest challenge in taking a narrative approach is knowing when to stop. Disease, disability, deprivation and death are not stories. They are facts (Launer 2001). Professionals who get carried away by narrative ideas to the point where they forget this, are not safe. Medical knowledge applied uncritically can lead to abuses of power, but pursuing narratives without a sense of reality can be literally fatal. Narrative ideas can help people question their own convictions, but no one should play postmodernist games with patients' lives.

The approach we now teach on the Tavistock Clinic training course, and hence the one proposed in this book, is an attempt to address these challenges. We have tried to do justice to a complex and sophisticated body of contemporary thought while also paying respect to the realities of life in the health service. We have tried to import some quite difficult concepts and techniques into primary care, without overloading busy clinicians with excessively abstract theories or jargon. The overriding intention is to present ideas in a way that is accessible and applicable. Where narrative ideas turn out to be worth adapting for everyday primary care, we have tried to do so. Where they turn out to be nonsensical in that setting, we have rejected them. Our aim is to bring them into primary care in a way that enables practitioners and hence empowers patients.

Systems, families, primary care and therapy: some definitions

A number of ideas in this book concern human systems like families, teams, professions or cultures. For a few years, we explicitly used the term 'systemic' in describing our approach. Systems theory and systemic family therapy have been fertile sources of new thinking for primary care and continue to be so (Fabb *et al.* 1997). However, 'systemic' is a problematical term. To some people it means nothing at all. Others are puzzled because they understand it only in the intravenous sense! Even for those who know something about family therapy, it can suggest a sectarian bias – something much narrower than we intend to convey (Shawver 2001). 'Narrative-based primary care' is a more accessible description of what we teach, and a more accurate one. It is therefore used throughout this book.

Inevitably, this book emphasises the family. This is not because of a belief that primary care is chiefly about the family, nor that it ought to be. There are many reasons why primary care should not necessarily be seen as synonymous with family practice (Toon 1995). However, the family is usually the most important context in people's lives and the one that most commonly makes itself known to primary care workers. 'Family' in this context has the widest possible meaning. It includes not just the nuclear family, but families in any of their other forms – including single parent families, gays and lesbians, adoptive or reconstituted families and those created by assisted conception. Its meaning extends to the remembered family, so that the isolated patient who has no immediate household or close living relatives will still produce stories in which the past or absent family plays a vital part. The family, however understood, is also part of a set of wider systems that help to determine its stories, including the community, the social class, the culture, the ethnic grouping and the religious faith.

Some of the book addresses only general practice. Most of it applies to a wide range of primary care professions. Self-evidently, some of the ideas apply only to particular professions rather than to all of them, although nearly everything in this book is designed to be of relevance to GPs, nurses and health visitors. Many of the ideas may be applicable to other areas of medicine and to other allied disciplines, but our experience so far has been only with primary care. Situated at the crossroads between the biological and biographical worlds, it seems the most natural place to try and develop a narrative approach (Gordon and Plamping 1996).

When the book refers to therapy, this does not imply formal sessions, nor working with whole families. One way of seeing primary care is as *ultra brief, ultra long therapy* (Launer 1994, 1996b). It is ultra brief because encounters are shorter than in any other setting. It is ultra long because relationships with patients can extend over immense periods of time, sometimes decades.

Even when this is not the case, the conversation may still extend over many episodes (Stange 2001). It is therapy in its literal sense: a form of healing.

An extract from the sources

This introduction and all the chapters in Part One include an extract from one of the theoretical sources of ideas in contemporary family therapy. These quotations do not necessarily represent the approach we propose, but they provide a background for the ideas, particularly for readers interested in the underlying theories that have informed this book.

> We live with each other, we work with each other and we love with each other. All this occurs in language ... The construction of meaning and understanding, the construction of human systems, is a constantly changing, creative and dynamic process. This view of human interconnectedness does not rely on a definition of perception and cognition that requires a representational or objective view of reality. Rather, this emerging position has at its core, the belief that reality is a social construction. We live and take action in a world that we define through our descriptive language in social intercourse with others ...
>
> Within this framework, there are no 'real' external entities, only communicating and languaging human individuals. There is only the process of the constantly evolving reality of language use. Thus there are no 'facts' to be known, no systems to be 'understood', and no patterns or regularities to be 'discovered'. This position demands that we give up the view of humankind as the 'knowers' of the essences of nature. It its place is substituted a view of humankind in continuing conversation.
>
> Conversation – language and communicative action – is simply part of the hermeneutic struggle to reach understanding with those with whom we are in contact. Said differently, language does not mirror nature; language creates the nature we know. Meaning and understanding do not exist prior to the utterances of language ... In this sense, understanding is always a process, 'on the way' and never fully achieved.

Harlene Anderson and Harold Goolishian (1988)

References

Anderson H and Goolishian H (1988) Human systems as linguistic systems: preliminary and evolving ideas about the implications for clinical theory. *Fam Proc.* **27**: 371–93.

Atkinson P (1995) *Medical Talk and Medical Work*. Sage, London.

Berger P and Luckmann T (1966) *The Social Construction of Reality*. Allen Lane, London.

Blumhagen D (1980) Hyper-tension: a folk illness with a medical name. *Cult Med Psychiatry*. 4: 197–227.

Bruner J (1986) *Actual Minds, Possible Worlds*. Harvard University Press, Cambridge, MA.

Bruner J (1990) *Acts of Meaning*. Harvard University Press, Cambridge, MA.

Calman KC (2001) A study of storytelling, humour and learning in medicine. *Clin Med*. 1: 227–9.

Cecchin G, Lane G and Ray W (1994) *The Cybernetics of Prejudices in the Practice of Psychotherapy*. Karnac, London.

Cole-Kelly K (1992) Illness stories and patient care in the family practice context. *Fam Med*. 24: 45–8.

Coulter A (1999) Paternalism or partnership? *BMJ*. **319**: 719–20.

Fabb WE, Chao DVK and Chan CSY (1997) The trouble with family medicine. *Fam Pract*. 14: 5–11.

Fine M and Turner J (1991) Tyranny and freedom: looking at ideas in the practice of family therapy. *Fam Proc*. **30**: 307–20.

Frank A (2001) *Acts of Witness: forms of engagement in illness*. Presentation at narrative based medicine conference, 3 September, Cambridge, UK.

Fruggeri L (1992) Therapeutic process as the social construction of change. In: S McNamee and K Gergen (eds) *Therapy as Social Construction*. Sage, London.

Geertz C (1973) *The Interpretation of Cultures*. Basic Books, New York.

Gergen KJ and Davis KE (eds) (1985) *The Social Construction of the Person*. Springer-Verlag, New York.

Goldner V (1985) Feminism and family therapy. *Fam Proc*. **24**: 31–47.

Gordon P and Plamping D (1996) Primary health care: its characteristics and potential. In: P Gordon and J Hadley (eds) *Extending Primary Care*. Radcliffe Medical Press, Oxford.

Greenhalgh T and Hurwitz B (1998) *Narrative Based Medicine: dialogue and discourse in clinical practice*. BMJ Books, London.

Hahn R and Gaines A (1985) *Physicians of Western Medicine*. Reidel, Dordrecht.

Harre R (ed) (1986) *The Social Construction of Emotions*. Blackwell, Oxford.

Heurtin-Roberts S (1993) 'High-pertension': the uses of a chronic folk illness for personal adaptation. *Soc Sci Med*. **37**: 285–94.

Hodgkin P (1996) Medicine, postmodernism, and the end of certainty. *BMJ*. **313**: 1568–9.

Hoffman L (1990) Constructing realities: an art of lenses. *Fam Proc*. **29**: 1–12.

Hunter KM (1991) *Doctors' Stories: the narrative structure of medical knowledge*. Princeton University Press, Oxford.

Kirmayer L (2001) *Narratives on Psychiatry*. Presentation at narrative based medicine conference, 3 September, Cambridge, UK.

Launer J (1994) Psychotherapy in the GP surgery: working with and without a secure therapeutic frame. *Br J Psychother*. **11**: 121–6.

Launer J (1996a) 'You're the doctor, Doctor!': is social constructionism a helpful stance in general practice consultations? *J Fam Ther*. **18**: 255–67.

Launer J (1996b) Toward systemic general practice. *Context*. **26**: 42–5.

Launer J (2001) Whatever happened to biology? Reconnecting family therapy with its evolutionary origins. *J Fam Ther*. **23**: 155–70.

Launer J (2002) The practice as an organisation. In: J Holmes and A Elder (eds) *Mental Health in Primary Care: a new approach*. Oxford University Press, Oxford.

Lock M and Gordon D (eds) (1988) *Biomedicine Examined*. Kluwer, Dordrecht.

Luepnitz D (1988) *The Family Interpreted: feminist theory in clinical practice*. Basic Books, New York.

Lupton D (1997) Consumerism, reflexivity and the medical encounter. *Soc Sci Med*. **45**: 373–81.

Lyotard J-F (1984) *The Post Modern Condition: a report on knowledge*. University of Minnesota Press, Minneapolis.

Mathers N and Rowland S (1997) General practice – a post-modern speciality? *Br J Gen Pract*. **47**: 177–9.

Mattingly C (1998) *Healing Dramas and Clinical Plots: the narrative structure of experience*. Cambridge University Press, Cambridge.

McNamee S and Gergen K (eds) (1992) *Therapy as Social Construction*. Sage, London.

McWhinney IR (1996) The importance of being different. *Br J Gen Pract*. **46**: 433–6.

Morris DB (1998) *Illness and Culture in the Postmodern Age*. University of California Press, California.

Muir Gray JA (1999) Post modern medicine. *Lancet*. **354**: 1550–3.

O'Brian C (1990) Family therapy with black families. *J Fam Ther*. **12**: 3–16.

Prest LA and Keller JF (1993) Spirituality and family therapy: spiritual beliefs, myths and metaphors. *J Marital Fam Ther*. **19**: 137–48.

Ricoeur P (1984) *Time and Narrative*, vol 1. University of Chicago Press, Chicago.

Riessman CK (1990) The strategic uses of narrative in the presentation of self and illness. *Soc Sci Med*. **30**: 1195–200.

Roberts G and Holmes J (eds) (1999) *Narrative in Psychiatry and Psychotherapy*. Oxford University Press, Oxford.

Shawver L (2001) If Wittgenstein and Lyotard could talk with Jack and Jill: towards post modern family therapy. *J Fam Ther*. **23**: 232–52.

Smith R (2001) Why are doctors so unhappy? *BMJ.* **322**: 1078.

Stange K (2001) The best of times and the worst of times. *Br J Gen Pract.* **51**: 963–6.

Toon P (1995) *What is Good General Practice?* Royal College of General Practitioners, London.

Walrond-Skinner S (1989) Spiritual dimensions and religious beliefs in family therapy. *J Fam Ther.* **11**: 47–67.

Wilson HJ (2000) The myth of objectivity: is medicine moving towards a social constructivist medical paradigm? *Fam Pract.* **17**: 203–9.

PART ONE

Practice

CHAPTER 1

The narrative practitioner at work

'My story is broken, can you help me fix it?'
Howard Brody (1994)

The purpose of this chapter is to give an overview of a narrative-based approach so that readers can gain a quick impression of what is on offer, and to consider what new ideas they are likely to discover from it. The overview is based on a description of one consultation between a man and his doctor. The doctor is attempting to work as a narrative practitioner.

The consultation is a compilation, drawn from several real ones to illustrate the approach. The description is interspersed with some commentary drawing attention to important themes. Many of these themes are discussed in more detail later in the book.

Key ideas in this chapter

- Narrative-based practitioners see their main task as helping the patient to develop a new story.
- This involves paying close attention to the patient's language and to the contexts that make sense of it.
- It also involves offering the patient choices about how to make use of the practitioner, and about how to proceed at each juncture in the consultation.
- Narrative-based practice does not need to be time-consuming. It can even save time by being focused and connected with the patient's needs.

Points to consider

- What are the distinctive features of this approach compared with other common approaches?
- How is it similar to what you already do and how is it different?
- What appeals to you, and what reservations or questions do you have?

The consultation

A patient walks into his GP's consulting room and starts to describe five different problems. It is a familiar moment, one that any GP or practice nurse would recognise as typical. As the patient goes through his list, the GP feels a mounting sense of stress. In her mind, she runs through a range of options she has learned from her former trainer, her colleagues and her years of experience.

Should she point out her own time pressures and say something about the limits of GP consultations? Would it be fair to ask the patient to choose just one problem to concentrate on? Perhaps it would help to comment on how overwhelmed she feels by the list and ask the patient if he too feels overwhelmed. Or is it best to let the patient speak without interruption, accepting the emotional burden and the delay to other patients?

Instead, she chooses a quite different strategy and asks: 'Do you think all these problems are separate ones or is there something that connects them?'

Generally, patients do not come into surgeries and clinics with stories that are well-formed and clearly articulated. Their initial narratives are much more likely to be hesitant, disjointed, fragmented, complicated or full of things that puzzle them. Whatever a new narrative does, it must provide a better kind of explanation and some coherence for what is happening to the patient. There may need to be a technical solution, but there will also need to be a story where some of the confusion is lessened, some of the fragments are united and some of the puzzles are solved. The patient who has been well treated in technical terms but cannot speak (or think) of a new story has not experienced any healing. In the particular consultation illustrated here, what chiefly guides the GP is the wish to help the patient towards a more coherent story.

The patient with five problems says: 'I don't think my problems are connected. I've just saved them up because it's hard to get to see you.'

The GP wonders for a moment if she should challenge the patient's explanation, perhaps with an inquiry about stress or an explanation about the appointment system. However, she decides it is better to accept his words at face value. She says: 'Is it all right if we start with the problem that's most important to you? Depending on how that goes, we may need to think later on about finding enough time for the other problems.'

Health professionals come to consultations with a rich set of prepared narratives in mind. These come from all kinds of sources, including the rules and regulations of the practice, their professional knowledge and training, personal experiences and beliefs. In any one encounter, the narrative in the clinician's mind may include such elements as '*I must keep good time*', '*I must appear interested*', '*I must be as good a GP as my trainer was*', '*I must practise good evidence-based medicine*', and so on.

The professional's narrative may be so dominant that it takes over the consultation completely. Patients then lose any chance to develop their own stories. Alternatively, practitioners can be aware of their own narratives, but hold these in abeyance. This is not to say they have to suppress or abolish them. There may well be occasions when they have to assert them: for example, when someone has serious symptoms or when a consultation has badly overrun. However, clinicians can use their own narratives with transparency, as the GP is trying to do here.

> From his five problems, the patient identifies tiredness as his most important problem. Having covered the routine ground of history taking (working pattern, sleeping habits and an enquiry about physical systems) the GP widens her scope of enquiry: 'Apart from yourself, who in your family do you think is most aware of your tiredness?'

Narratives never exist in isolation. They are forged in relationships with friends and families, contacts and acquaintances, colleagues and communities. To make sense of any narrative, and to provide an opportunity for it to change, we have to make some enquiry into the densely populated background of what is being said. Pursuing a narrative in primary care inevitably means pursuing an interest in the family. This is not because families in any sense 'cause' problems, or because it is the family's responsibility to solve them. It is because most people create their stories largely in family conversations. In addition, illness nearly always has an impact on the family – whether this means having someone at home with flu, or the huge disruption that occurs when a parent or a child is seriously ill or disabled (Altschuler 1997; Altschuler and Dale 1999).

Professionals have families too, in both a literal and a metaphorical sense. The literal family may be present in all sorts of subtle ways in the consultation: in memories, habits, assumptions, expectations or as photos on the desk. The metaphorical family consists of the partnership, the practice, the profession, and all the present and past systems that have contributed to the stories in practitioners' minds, and to their preferences in the way they like stories to go. Thus, it may be helpful to regard every consultation as an intersection of two families – the practitioner's and the patient's – as represented in the minds and narratives of both. While both may often need to be discussed, it is nearly always the patient's family that needs to be brought into the conversation.

> After a few more minutes the patient and GP have established that the tiredness dates from the death of the patient's father-in-law. His wife has

been sunk in grief and he has had to take on most of the domestic duties. The GP suggests that his wife should attend for a consultation, either by herself or with her husband. The patient says he has already suggested this but his wife is adamant she will get through her bereavement on her own. She has evidently had previous encounters with a counsellor but found these intrusive and upsetting. She generally has no truck with 'talking things through'.

   The GP toys with a number of possible interventions, including a sympathetic phone call to the wife or sending a reassuring message of invitation through the husband. Rejecting either of these courses, she asks: 'If your wife doesn't change her mind about coming herself, what's the most helpful thing I can do in relation to your own tiredness?'

At almost any moment in a consultation, the practitioner has the option of taking charge: for example by 'spelling out the rules', by taking unilateral action, by deciding what is best for the patient or by foreclosing the encounter. However, there is nearly always an alternative. It is to hand over the threads of the story, or the narrative lead, to the patient. The GP here has done exactly that. Rather than challenging the realities of the patient's life, she acknowledges them. Instead of deciding 'the best way forward', she asks what use the patient wants to make of her. In effect, she continually asks not just *'How are you today?'* but also *'Who am I today – for you?'*

> In response to his GP's question, the patient says he can largely deal with his own tiredness but he would be reassured by a checkup. He says he has found it helpful today just to have an opportunity to talk about his wife's bereavement and how much he has had to support her. He feels certain that he can see her through this difficult phase in her life if the doctor can lay to rest his own anxieties about his health. He wonders if the doctor can also address the other four problems that have been bothering him (a skin blemish, a painful wrist, ear wax and a toenail problem) during the checkup. The GP accepts his judgement. She suggests a further appointment for the following week.

Reviewing this consultation, one thing is perhaps worth noticing above all others. It is the doctor's attentiveness to language. Wherever possible, she follows the exact words of her patient rather than her own speculations about those words. When he says his five problems are unconnected, she accepts this. When he says his wife would not consider coming, the doctor pursues alternatives rather than challenging him. She treats language not as a mere starting point for her own chain of associations but as an utterly authoritative guide for the conduct of the interview. Her consulting style is not driven by the attempt to make one single decision – or five separate ones – in order to solve the patient's problems. It is driven by language, and by a series of micro-decisions about how to proceed in the conversation itself. Each of these micro-decisions is shared with the patient. The doctor's main focus is not on producing diagnoses or treatments (although these may play a part in the next consultation). It is on producing a shared new narrative.

As a result, in a short space of time, she and the patient are able to put together a story that is an improvement on the opening one, satisfies the patient for the time being, and fits with her own understanding of her role and its limitations.

> At the end of her consultation with the tired man, the GP reflects that the outcome is perhaps not very different to what it might have been if she had conducted it more conventionally. But she has a sense that the man has participated more fully in the way the consultation was constructed. She hopes he may have experienced it as therapeutic, and makes a mental note to ask him next time if anything that happened in this consultation was particularly helpful. She feels less stressed than she expected, and she has almost kept to time.

Suggested exercises

- After a consultation, compare the final story with the initial one that the patient brought. How was it different? How far was it a medical one and what other elements did it have?
- After a consultation, try to recall how many people or organisations were mentioned in it.
- After a consultation, recall how you managed limitations of time or resources, or indicated them.
- In any consultation, pay attention to the first juncture when you asked a question. Afterwards, think about why you chose that juncture. What then happened? What other questions could you have asked? What might have happened if you had?
- In another consultation, try to pay attention to the first two or three questions in the same way.

An extract from the sources

We may consider narration to be a reciprocal exercise, consisting both of the act of telling the story and the act of responding to it. In this mutual, interactive approach, the physician does not simplistically 'take a history' but is also prepared to see the patient narrative grow and change over time, and to participate in that process. In this interpretation, the act of co-creation of patient narrative must be mutually negotiated between physician and patient. Such an approach assumes the intrinsic value of patient narrative, although it does not conform to biomedical rules and formats, and does not attempt to dismiss this narrative once the essential 'biomedical' aspects have been extracted . . .

The physician also has a responsibility to challenge automatic or conventional elements of the patient's story, in effect, to say to the patient, 'it seems to me there is much more to tell here'. In this guise, the physician's responsibility is to help the patient's tale gain momentum and depth, to draw out the story in hiding. In a similar vein, the physician commits to scrutinising the patient's story in order to find new meanings that may more accurately reflect the reality of the storyteller and, in doing so, help the storyteller see where the story wants to go . . .

The physician can also attempt to recognise and/or encourage conditions that facilitate the creation of meaning during the process of patient narrative. In eliciting a patient narrative, the physician must encourage the patient to be emotionally engaged in his or her story, in other words to acknowledge fears, hopes, and expectations . . . Finally, to facilitate a meaningful patient story, the physician must help patients take the risk of confessing those aspects of their story that are confusing and full of gaps. When we demand certainty, patients oblige with fictive information that conforms to our logico-scientific criteria, but distorts the patient's reality. When we allow ambiguity and mystery their place in the treatment room, patients have permission to offer narratives with those qualities as well.

Joanna Shapiro (1993)

References

Altschuler J (1997) *Working with Chronic Illness and Disability.* With contributions from Barbara Dale and John Byng-Hall. Macmillan, Basingstoke.

Altschuler J and Dale B (1999) On being an ill parent. *Clin Child Psychol Psychiatry.* 4: 23–37.

Brody H (1994) 'My story is broken: can you help me fix it?' Medical ethics and the joint construction of narrative. *Lit Med.* 13: 79–92.

Shapiro J (1993) The use of narrative in the doctor–patient encounter. *Fam Sys Med.* 11: 47–53.

CHAPTER 2

Concepts

'Not knowing means humility about what one knows. In effect, a therapist is more interested in learning what a client has to say than in pursuing, telling, validating or promoting his or her knowledge or preoccupations.'
Harlene Anderson (1997)

This chapter presents a framework of concepts that can help people to take a narrative-based approach.

Most people embarking on a narrative approach seem to find it useful to learn a conceptual framework at the outset. It emphasises the crucial differences from other approaches. It serves as a simple summary of complex ideas. It can also provide a set of mental prompts for people when practising a narrative approach. However, different people respond to the concepts in different ways. Some people are profoundly struck by them. They feel as if they are opening up a window on a quite new way of looking at their work. For others, the concepts seem 'just like common sense', although they may find it affirming to hear about ideas they understand instinctively but have not previously read about.

One possible description of the framework is that it is 'a map of therapeutic intuition'. This description draws attention to one essential characteristic of this framework, or indeed of any other: it can only map out a state of mind and emotion, it can never fully convey it. It is itself a 'story'. Each person who enters a dialogue with it will turn it into a further, unique story.

Key ideas in this chapter

- Family therapy offers a number of key concepts that are useful in everyday primary care. Most of these are based on familiar words but used in specific ways.
- The fundamental reorientation for taking a narrative approach involves seeing the world in terms of circular processes rather than linear ones.
- It also involves seeing the consultation as a shared act of creation between someone with a problem and some else with a body of expert knowledge and skills.

Points to consider

- What do these concepts contribute to your understanding of a narrative approach?
- How far are these ideas familiar and obvious, and what is new about them for you?
- How might you apply them?
- What problems do you anticipate if you tried to put them into practice? How could you overcome these?
- How useful do you find it to have a conceptual framework? Do you currently use an alternative one (perhaps from another published source, or one of your own)?

Narrative concepts and primary care

Some concepts from family therapy work well in primary care. Others do not. Over time, we have found that the ones that work best are simple, intuitive and generally free of jargon. Six main concepts seem to be particularly helpful. Conveniently, they all begin with the letter 'c'. The six concepts are:

- conversations
- curiosity
- circularity
- contexts
- co-creation
- caution.

Although most of these words are very familiar ones from everyday English usage, they are each used with a particular meaning in the context of narrative practice, and these meanings are covered here. Each of these concepts has been extensively discussed in the family therapy literature. This chapter presents them in a way designed to bring out their relevance for primary care, but they are referenced so that readers who wish to can explore their theoretical origins.

This chapter and many in the rest of this book are illustrated by a number of cases. These are mostly taken from stories that have been told or written by people on our courses. (A small minority of stories in the book are from the author's own practice.) Every story, here and elsewhere, has been heavily disguised to prevent anyone accidentally recognising the patients or the practitioners involved.

Conversations

As Chapter 1 illustrated, a narrative approach sees conversations in a special way: not as a vehicle for treatment but as the treatment itself. This is different from seeing 'the doctor as treatment' or empathy alone as crucial. It means seeing the conversational process itself as therapy. It involves moving away from the idea of 'problem solving' and towards the idea of 'problem dissolution', through the creation of new stories (Andersen 1992). The main way that problem dissolution occurs in the course of medical conversations is by inviting patients to consider their problems in alternative ways. The invitation may come in the suggestion that something can be given a medical name and a treatment. But it may also come through a suggestion that the problem can be thought of in different ways, in a wider context, or with a new form of words. Instead of being a fixer or an adviser, the clinician becomes a questioner and a proposer of reframed stories.

This way of looking at consultations puts both the participants – the patient and the clinician – on a level field. It can absolve clinicians from the sense of total responsibility for what happens – a sense of responsibility that so often oppresses them. Within the context of primary care, a further advantage is that it removes the apparently pressing need to produce 'endings' on each occasion. From a narrative point of view, no story really ever ends: it simply evolves.

Taking conversations seriously means taking language seriously. This in turn means applying a disciplined attentiveness to the exact story as it is, and tracking the patient's language exactly, as the doctor did in the previous chapter. It means making enquiry into the words that have actually been said, and not into what one merely thought the patient meant – let alone into some quite extraneous matter that happens to have come into one's mind. The American family therapist Harold Goolishian apparently used to sum up this attitude with the advice: '*Don't listen to what patients mean, listen to what they say*'. Much of the technical advice later in this book is concerned with how to develop and apply such attentiveness.

Curiosity (and neutrality)

Therapists often discuss what makes an encounter therapeutic. There is now a consensus that the common denominator here is a certain kind of curiosity (Cecchin 1987). This is not intrusive curiosity (as in 'curiosity killed the cat'.) It means a focused and committed interest – an interest that can move the conversation forward from Story A to Story B. It is the opposite of paternalism or stereotypical questioning. Also, curiosity of this kind is not just something intellectual. It involves emotional engagement as well, so that there is an identification both with patients' feelings and with their understanding of those feelings.

The following case example shows effective curiosity in action in one GP's work, in a way that will be very familiar to many readers.

Being curious about Sam M

Sam M is 35, divorced and has been registered with me for five years. He first reported symptoms of excessive fatigue the year after he registered. The following year he then had a bout of gastroenteritis that lasted for two weeks. Following this he continued to have recurrent diarrhoea and abdominal pain. He also felt unwell and tired all the time. Blood tests and stool culture were all normal. As he was no better after two months I referred him for a gastroenterological opinion. They made a diagnosis of post-enteric irritable bowel syndrome after a negative barium enema. Medication and high-fibre diet produced little improvement in his symptoms. From September he began to work from home for some of the time, although I did not learn about this until later. In March, he was reviewed by the gastroenterologist and started on amitriptyline. By April he felt too unwell to work and requested a medical certificate.

At this point I felt I really needed to be more interested in this patient. I started seeing him regularly and giving him longer to talk. He has a responsible and demanding job. He said he felt unable to return to work as he was still having unpredictable bouts of diarrhoea. I asked if he thought he would be able to get better if he did not have to return to work. It became apparent he was ambivalent in his feelings about his job. He described his boss as 'a workaholic' and said he felt obliged to be the same, working long hours and weekends. As a result he had lost friends and given up interests. Since he had been off work his boss had been phoning frequently asking when he was returning.

I asked about his family and he said he was close to his parents, who had been concerned for several years about his workload. He was previously married for a couple of years and had no children. Since his marriage broke down he hasn't been in a relationship and says he just threw himself into his work.

I've seen him three times now, for about 15 minutes each time. He has decided to resign from his present job and when he is better look for a less stressful part-time job. He is planning a holiday with his brother. Since telling his boss he will not be returning, he has begun to feel better with more energy and fewer bowel symptoms. He is still seeing me regularly and I hope his physical symptoms will continue to improve now he has resolved his dilemma about his job.

A crucial aspect of therapeutic curiosity is *neutrality*. The term neutrality, as used by family therapists, is not the same as a lack of opinion, or of emotion, or of moral engagement. It is, first, neutrality in the sense of being able to focus on the task – namely to help people with their own stories as they see them and not as you expect them to be. It implies a tolerance of different points of view. It may also show itself as a consulting stance that studiously demonstrates tolerance of several different points of view being expressed at the same time by different family members (Palazzoli Selvini *et al.* 1980).

There is also a wider meaning to neutrality. It is neutrality in the face of all facts. This may take the form of setting aside a strong belief that someone's illness is mainly a physical one or, conversely, that it is mainly a psychological one. It may even mean setting aside the notion that an illness exists – or indeed does not exist! The acid test will be whether the words and descriptions on offer are helpful to the patient. This expanded definition of neutrality has been defined as an intentional stance of 'not knowing' (Anderson and Goolishian 1992). The stance of 'not knowing' is defined in the epigraph at the beginning of this chapter, from the therapist Harlene Anderson.

People commonly misunderstand the idea of neutrality in a number of different ways. It is worth looking at these misunderstandings because they often inhibit people's confidence in developing a neutral stance. First, neutrality does *not* mean forgetting one's professional role as a medical expert with a recognised corpus of knowledge (Efran and Clarfield 1992; Graham *et al.* 1995). However, it does involve recognising that, for a variety of reasons, this knowledge may not connect at all with the story of the other person in the room.

Second, neutrality does not mean setting aside moral standards (Glaser 1991). It does not require practitioners to forsake their beliefs, or the values that inspire their work. It certainly should not stop people from taking action in cases where the patient's health is seriously at risk. The aim of neutrality is not to disable action but to pursue a fuller understanding of the problem. (Further issues concerning neutrality are discussed from a theoretical perspective in Chapter 16.)

Therapists often quote the adage: '*the only person you can change is yourself*'. Remembering this is a good way to hold on to curiosity and neutrality. It invites professionals to be curious not only about their patients but about themselves too: why they have become stuck, or determined to convince the patient of a particular truth, or annoyed if they cannot do so. It reminds professionals that they are unlikely to help patients to develop a new story unless they have tried to understand themselves dispassionately in the consultation and have retained the capacity to become neutral towards their own story of what is going on – and to change it.

Circularity

Circularity lies at the heart of the way family therapists understand their work (Watzlawick *et al.* 1967). It is a view of the world as an infinite pattern of interactions. In some ways it is a view that is particularly difficult for healthcare professionals to take on board, schooled as they are in traditional 'linear' ideas such as the clinching diagnosis and the ideal treatment. Yet in another way, it is a very familiar idea in the medical world: think of those immense, vivid and complex diagrams of the Krebs cycle, full of feedback loops. Think of them, furthermore (as one should) not as something static but as an endless, three-dimensional dance without perceptible beginning or end, held in a tension between homoeostatic tendencies and evolutionary potential, and you have both an ideal example and a perfect metaphor for circularity in human interactions.

In terms of work between primary care professionals and patients, and the story making that goes on between them, circularity is an essential concept. It reminds us that the stories we participate in do not have beginnings and endings except in so far as we choose to punctuate them into encounters and consultations to suit our own pragmatic needs. It also reminds us that the stories made up between two people are the merest fraction of the stories that surround the two people involved, let alone the stories that surround those – and so on 'ad infinitum'.

How can a creative sense of circularity be brought into the consulting room? The most important way is by continually following feedback in the conversation, as demonstrated by the doctor in Chapter 1. By paying respect to language, by tracking it as she does and responding precisely to each response, she is herself modelling a circular process rather than a linear one (Palazzoli Selvini *et al.* 1980).

Another way of bringing circularity into the room is by the use of what family therapists call 'circular questions' (Penn 1983). The term is perhaps unfortunate as it suggests a process that goes nowhere, and nothing could be further from its true intention. Circular questions are in fact any questions that reflect or transmit a view of the world functioning according to circular principles, as opposed to linear ones. They may be questions that expand the view of the problem by inviting the patient to place it in a wider context of family relationships or time. They may be questions that literally circle around different family members as an interviewer carefully poses questions in turn to explore how each person affects others in the family dance. Circular questions are discussed in greater detail in the next chapter, and at a number of points in the book.

Using such techniques, the aim is to move both practitioner and patient away from fixed ideas of single causes and simple effects, of unchangeable problems and of over-concrete diagnoses. This can lead to stories that may be far more polyphonic, subtle, complex and interesting, and offer more potential for change, than the old ones. The following story from a GP is an example.

Asking Maria C circular questions

A patient called Maria C came to see me. She had unfortunately developed a basal cell carcinoma on one of her eyelids, and the surgeon who had initially removed it had made an unsightly excision. She arranged to be seen by another surgeon and she was offered a wide excision and a skin graft. She wanted to see me to talk over her options.

When she came to see me, she referred to the appearance of the skin graft. She tried to make light of it, but I was quite shocked at the disfigurement she had endured. We talked about the way other people in her life were reacting to the sight of the obvious facial deformity.

I started to ask her some circular questions: who, in her family, was most worried about her condition? She replied without hesitation that it was her father, who is widowed and lives back in Italy. I asked her some more questions: what did this cancer mean to her and to the other important people in her life? She explained that she was the only child. There was hefty pressure on her to go back and live with her father and look after him, which would have been 'the done thing' in Italian families, where an unmarried daughter was expected to care for parents for the full duration of their lives. Her family were counselling her against getting any further surgery, and in her mind this was connected with their wish for her to be 'a proper daughter' and look after her father as her first priority.

Using questions in this way, I learned a great deal about her family's interactions, as well as beliefs about her illness. This helped her to look at her own confusion as to whether she wished to care for her family, or whether she wished her family to care for her, as she had now suffered an illness. She told me that she had enormous difficulty in getting on with her father and could not contemplate living with him. She also felt guilty, as she had pursued a career which evoked disapproval from the whole family.

I remember this consultation because I was struck how this kind of questioning gave me an additional resource at my disposal. It helped me and my patient to look at the implications of the options on offer. It was also such a strong feeling of 'bringing the family into the room', even though only a single member was with me.

Contexts

Everything we say always has multiple contexts. For a story to evolve, participants need to share an understanding of the weighting and the implications of the words that are being used. It is usually impossible to understand any utterance fully without an accurate understanding of its main contexts, and indeed the relationship between the various contexts (Cronen *et al.* 1985).

Patients are surrounded by multiple contexts. They come to consultations with stories that constructed in previous conversations with families, friends, workmates or healthcare professionals. These in turn are embedded in history and geography, in lifelong personal and family experience, in gender and class relations, in interest groups and in faith communities. The most effective way of developing narrative is therefore to make an enquiry into such contexts, especially into past encounters with the health service, and the family and work contexts. This is demonstrated in the two cases above.

Practitioners bring their own contexts too. These include their training, traditions, regulations and professional codes of practice. They also include a wide range of personal contexts that may be very similar to the patients' – or entirely different.

When patients and practitioners converse, they are influenced by all sorts of professional contexts related to the work setting itself: booking systems, appointment lengths, the ways in which the primary care team operates and so on. They are affected by their previous encounters, and by how well the participants already know each other. Patients do not talk to doctors in the same way they do to nurses or to pharmacists. Nor do they talk to either of these in the way they talk to their greengrocers or their lovers.

From a narrative point of view, one of the most important contexts for primary care is that it is a medical context. This leads some patients to feel that they 'ought' to bring physical symptoms even when they are partly or wholly aware that these are not the chief source of their distress. It also puts pressure on practitioners to offer certain conventional kinds of response rather than other, perhaps more imaginative ones. However, there is another, more positive side to this too. It means that there is a safe setting for carrying out a whole range of conventional but helpful medical activities (physical examination, prescriptions and so on) often at considerable speed, without these being continually brought into question.

When consultations fail, it is often because important contexts have not been noticed, or defined, or discussed. As a result, the new story may be even more unsatisfactory or even more of a muddle than the old one. Many unsatisfactory or puzzling encounters in primary care can be freed up by talking about the professional and social contexts that surround them; '*bringing the context into the room'*. Examples are limitless, but people appear to find the following questions useful.

- 'Before I can answer your question, it will help me to ask a few questions to try and pin things down ...'
- 'I'd like to check you over physically because that may help me understand what's causing this ...'
- 'Since we've got only limited time, is there anything you think it's particularly important for me to concentrate on?'
- 'Is there anything you're hoping I might say or do that's different from other doctors you've seen?'
- 'You come from a different country to this one. What do you think your own doctor at home would say about this, or do about it?'
- 'I'd be interested to know what you made of that experience as a black person. Would you see racial discrimination as a possible factor?'
- 'How do you think things would be different if you were seeing a doctor who was a woman?'
- 'Had you come today mainly hoping for reassurance, or a diagnosis, or was it something else?'
- 'Who else do you think you might turn to for help with this problem?'
- 'If we can't sort this problem out between the two of us, what do you think you might do next?'

Co-creation

One concept unites all the others that have been introduced so far. It is the 'co-creation' of stories (sometimes termed 'co-construction'). A narrative approach sees conversations as a process in which two people are interweaving their original stories so that they can jointly create a new one (Parry 1991).

In an ordinary conversation, two people simply have to talk to each other without any particular degree of self-consciousness. However, in a healthcare setting the roles of the two participants in the act of co-creation are not the same. The patient brings a problem and the clinician is paid to help with it. The professional therefore has a dual role – both as a participant and as someone who has to monitor the progress of the new story. One useful way to frame this dual role is to see the professional as an 'observer-participant' in the act of co-creation (Cox 2001).

Being an observer in a consultation has been described as 'going up on the ceiling and looking down at yourself and the patient'. Being an observer-participant is therefore like being up on the ceiling and down in the room at the same time. This stance is probably essential for narrative-based practice. It means cultivating the ability to contribute to the new story while at the same time tracking its progress through one's own and the patient's contributions, and the interaction between the two. It also means taking into account the complex and multilayered social contexts in which consultations take place, while still remaining emotionally engaged. It therefore means taking responsibility for restraint in the use of professional power: for example, not imposing narratives that reflect the view of a particular gender, ethnic group or profession.

Many readers might recognise that they already work in this way, although they might use different words to describe it. However, naming the professional role as being that of 'observer-participant' seems to help people to become both more involved and more detached in the process of co-creating stories. This is not the paradox it sounds. People become more involved in the sense of staying close to what their patients are telling them or asking them. They become more detached in the sense of watching the effect of their own proffered questions or stories on the patient, and through their increased ability to change these questions or stories in response to what they hear. This is particularly helpful when trying to balance the 'grand narrative' of medicine with the patient's personal narrative, in order to co-create a better story.

Caution

One GP told this tale.

The cautionary tale of Andrew H

A 25-year-old man, Andrew H, newly registered with the practice, consulted me about pain in his shoulders. He explained he had been lifting furniture and he asked for painkillers. It seemed likely that his shoulder pain was a trivial strain and I found myself far more interested in his look of distress. I asked him why he had been lifting furniture. He told me that he had just left his first job as he could not cope with the stress any more, and moved back with his mother. I invited him back as I wanted to have a discussion of his family background.

He duly returned for another appointment and I found out about his family. He was the youngest of four children, but his parents had divorced. The father had not kept in touch with the family. He had always felt that his mother didn't like him, perhaps because he was born when the marriage was already failing, and left him out of things, favouring the three siblings. Now back in the family home having failed to stay away, he felt that his mother thought worse of him than ever. His mother was not in touch with her own parents who were in Scotland, as Andrew thought his father was too.

At the end of the consultation I felt that I had understood much more about Andrew and his problems. However, I noticed that he looked more unhappy and I asked how he had found the family discussion. He bravely replied: 'I think you are wasting my time doctor – I don't want to talk about my family. It isn't any use.' I felt disconcerted by this and I offered another appointment, to discuss whatever he wished on the next occasion.

He did not come back. He saw one of my partners, who has spent more time concentrating on his shoulders and has fixed up some physiotherapy. This case helped me to understand the importance of setting the context for dialogue outside the usual expectations of the GP–patient interaction. By extending the doctor–patient dialogue to family matters, I risked using my power to intrude into personal areas which the patient might rather keep private. Since this experience I have tried to offer a discussion of family background to a patient as an option of potential interest and use to both of us, just as a physical investigation like an x-ray might be.

Learners who become excessively fired by narrative ideas can start to behave as if they were formal therapists. This is inappropriate. Patients do not come to primary care for formal therapy, and can find it alienating. Besides, the time is too short for formal therapy and the social setting quite inappropriate for this. Although most learners do go through an unsettling period when they are adapting to a new way of seeing their work (and sometimes their world), it will usually not help them if they devalue or abandon everything they have learned before. The most inspired people are often those who have been able to make their own synthesis – their own new professional narrative – by incorporating a number of different approaches into a narrative framework.

Suggested exercises

- Review a consultation. What contexts did you enquire into? What other contexts might you ask about on another occasion?
- How far was the final story 'co-created' with the patient? Are there things you could have said or asked to make it more so?
- Choose one of the 'six Cs'. Think about it during a consultation (or take each concept in turn, one per consultation). How well does the concept

fit what is going on? Does it suggest any new ways of saying things or of asking questions?

- When time is not too pressing, try to observe your own chain of questioning during a consultation. How far is it led by habit and how far does it follow the patient's language?
- After a consultation, jot down some questions you would like to ask the patient the next time.

An extract from the sources

In order for new stories – or new relation between stories – to consolidate themselves in the therapeutic conversation, they must evolve from and yet contain elements of the old, 'familiar' stories. The transformed stories are usually a recombination of the components of the old story to which new elements – characters, plot, logic, moral order – have been introduced either by the therapist, by the patient or by the family as a result of, for example, circular questioning, and they are consolidated by all the participants through therapeutic conversation ... A new story that is too different from the old story will not be recognised by the clients as theirs, and it will simply be rejected as not pertinent. However, if a new story is too similar to the old one, it will not 'hold' because the old story tends to reconstitute itself through its many attachments to the material world that is already familiar to the clients ...

Stories about problems, symptoms, or conflicts – the thousand and one stories about answers to the question 'What brought you to the consultation' or 'What can I do for you?' – are organised around characters and their many attributes, relationships and vicissitudes; plots and events, and the degree of agency of the participants; settings and the weight they have on events; the ethical corollaries or unavoidable consequences for the participants. In addition, stories can be told in a fashion in which the story teller ... is portrayed as protagonist, bystander, witness, or interpreter of events, and with varying degrees of competency and reliability ... However, it should be understood that most of these dimensions are inextricably connected, and that a shift in any one of them affects each of the others. In turn, any shift in a story may effect the story's relative position within the complex network of narratives that constitute individual and familial reality.

Carlos Sluzki (1992)

References

Andersen T (1992) Reflections on reflecting with families. In: S McNamee and K Gergen (eds) *Therapy as Social Construction*. Sage, London.

Anderson H (1997) *Conversation, Language and Possibilities*. Basic Books, New York.

Anderson H and Goolishian H (1992) The client is the expert: a not-knowing approach to therapy. In: S McNamee and K Gergen (eds) *Therapy as Social Construction*. Sage, London.

Cecchin G (1987) Hypothesising, circularity, and neutrality revisited: an invitation to curiosity. *Fam Proc.* **26**: 405–13.

Cox K (2001) Hearing what the patient is thinking: implications for care and education. *Educ for Health.* **14**: 5–10.

Cronen VE, Pearce WB and Tomm K (1985) A dialectical view of personal change. In: KJ Gergen and KE Davis (eds) *The Social Construction of the Person*. Springer-Verlag, New York.

Efran JS and Clarfield LE (1992) Constructionist therapy: sense and nonsense. In: S McNamee and K Gergen (eds) *Therapy as Social Construction*. Sage, London.

Glaser D (1991) Neutrality and child abuse: a useful juxtaposition? *Hum Sys.* **2**: 149–60.

Graham H, Launer J, Mayer R and Young V (1995) Neutrality and medical responsibility: a debate around the treatment of asthma. *Context.* **25**: 43–5.

Palazzoli Selvini M, Boscolo L, Cecchin G and Prata G (1980) Hypothesising-circularity-neutrality: three guidelines for the conductor of the session. *Fam Proc.* **19**: 3–12.

Parry A (1991) A universe of stories. *Fam Proc.* **30**: 37–54.

Penn P (1983) Circular questioning. *Fam Proc.* **21**: 267–80.

Sluzki C (1992) Transformations, a blueprint for narrative changes in therapy. *Fam Proc.* **31**: 217–30.

Watzlawick T, Bavelas JB and Jackson DD (1967) *Pragmatics of Human Communication*. WW Norton, New York.

CHAPTER 3

Techniques

'Any time you speak in order to invite others to speak, so you can listen, this is talking-in-order-to-listen ... When you listen in order to talk, you listen for something to criticise, or for a way to insert your own opinions.'
Lois Shawver (2001)

This chapter looks at some specific techniques for exploring and creating narratives. These techniques are ways of putting into action the concepts described in Chapter 2. Although the techniques all derive from family therapy, they are presented here in a way that results from being honed down over several years, in order to address the needs of people working in primary care. They all coincide in some ways with techniques that many primary care practitioners may use by instinct, or on the basis of experience. The principal advantage of presenting them systematically may be that they provide a naming system – a 'story' – for things that many clinicians do every day. They therefore offer a vocabulary to help people with further skills development.

Key ideas in this chapter

- There are some specific consulting techniques that can often help patients to develop helpful new stories. These techniques can be learned and practised.
- Some of these techniques involve asking questions in particularly creative or imaginative ways. Others involve taking a stance that passes power over to the patient.
- One of the most important aspects of narrative technique is a constant process of reflection on what is happening in the conversation. This in turn can lead to more effective questions and comments.

Points to consider

- How do these techniques resemble what you already do?
- What ideas do they give you about expanding your technical repertoire? How feasible does this seem?
- What obstacles might you face? Who else could help you address them?
- Is narrative-based primary care turning into a coherent 'story' for you? What is still missing? What would you need to know for the story to make better sense?

Conversations inviting change: techniques for narrative development

As the two previous chapters have shown, questions are absolutely central in narrative technique, just as they are in conventional history taking. The difference is that narrative-based questions – especially so-called 'circular' questions – are not used just to establish facts but in order to develop the story. Wherever possible, questioning is done by picking up words or phrases that the patient has just used and seeking to 'unpack' them. This involves clarifying their meaning, but also seeing where they lead in terms of other ideas – especially ideas that the patient has not considered until the question is asked.

Another way of describing this kind of questioning is that one is always looking for 'the cutting edge' of the story, the single idea that suggests the possibility of new understanding for both practitioner and patient, and of change. The overall purpose of questioning is to take the patient from familiar, well-rehearsed territory into new directions that may offer a more helpful story about what is going on. This approach to consultations is sometimes referred to as 'interventive interviewing' (Tomm 1987a, b 1988). However, it may be better to think of it in terms of 'conversations inviting change'. This suggests something less assertive on the part of the practitioner and more participatory for the patient.

Like Chapter 1, this chapter is based on one illustrative consultation, this time between a patient and a practice nurse. However, it is presented in the form of a transcript. The transcript has been conflated from a number of actual consultations in order to demonstrate different techniques. The techniques discussed are:

- exploring differences and connections
- hypothesising
- circular questioning

- strategising
- sharing power
- reflection
- finding a good new story.

The consultation is presented in short extracts, interspersed with a commentary discussing each technique. The techniques are discussed discretely, but the nurse's comments and questions show how in practice they are all used in conjunction with each other – as inseparable aspects of 'conversations inviting change'. (To get the most out of this chapter, readers may find it helpful to read the whole consultation through first. The complete transcript appears at the end of the chapter.)

Exploring differences and connections

Patient: I've got a sore throat.
Nurse: Tell me about it.
Patient: I'm surprised how painful an ordinary sore throat can be.

Every narrative contains hints and openings that make it different from any other narrative that has ever taken place. The patient who presents with an 'ordinary' sore throat will almost inevitably use a word or phrase that marks his or her experience of it as unique. Looking for difference means paying attention to that unique moment, and enquiring into it.

Nurse: I wonder why that is. Is it quite unusual for you to have this kind of thing?
Patient: It's not just that. I'm concerned the pain has lasted so long.

If difference is on one side of the coin, connections are on the other. A narrative is made up of connections that are personal to that particular patient. Often they are signalled quite delicately – perhaps because of fear or through embarrassment – but the signals can be amplified, as shown here.

Nurse: That's not uncommon, but if it's your first it can be a bit of a shock. Are there any particular concerns you have about it?
Patient: Well, maybe I'm being a complete hypochondriac, but I've heard that heart trouble can make your throat hurt.

To explore connections, the practitioner has to follow the patient's feedback not just once but through a series of exchanges. For many clinicians in primary care, this is an odd experience when they first try it. It may feel like an interrogation or something that is at risk of careering off into an infinite chain of associations. Yet it usually turns out that the chain is quite a short one.

> Nurse: Your symptoms sound quite different, but are there other things making you worry it's your heart?
> Patient: Apart from my throat, nothing else is hurting.

A number of things are worth noting at this point. One is that the nurse is already combining good narrative technique with sound biomedical enquiry. She is not ruling out the possibility that there may be other, significant physical symptoms that the patient has not yet disclosed. Also, she is careful to place herself in the picture as an expert by saying that the sore throat does not sound like heart disease. This kind of comment, grounding the inquiry in professional normality, is essential so that this patient is not left feeling that he is in the hands of an intrusive questioner with no professional views of her own.

Hypothesising

Hypothesising is a very familiar process in the world of medicine. The GP who sees a patient with abdominal pain will carry out a very sophisticated process of testing and rejecting hypotheses while taking a history. What is different about hypothesising and narratives is that it addresses not just physical diagnoses but the whole area of human behaviour and relationships (Palazzoli Selvini et al. 1980).

> Nurse: Is there any other reason you might worry about heart disease?
> Patient: Yes, my father had a lot of heart trouble and he died from a heart attack last year. He was only 49.

If you consider the nurse being depicted in the vignette here, she has already pursued two hypotheses.

- Although this seems like a trivial problem, this patient thinks there is something serious going on.
- His worries about heart disease have a specific context that helps to explain them.

Of course, everyone working in primary care spends a great deal of their time testing hypotheses like these, with or without taking an explicitly narrative stance. This is often done at a subliminal level or on the basis of previous experience. Yet there are at least two good reasons for making the process explicit in one's own mind, especially at the learning stage.

- Identifying your hypotheses as you go along can make you more aware of when you hit on a productive line of questioning and when you do not.
- Cultivating the discipline of noticing your hypotheses, and of testing them with questions and following feedback, makes it easier to drop hypotheses that clearly prove to be of no interest or help to the patient.

Circular questioning

Like hypothesising, the process of asking questions is one that comes naturally to people who work in primary care. That is a significant advantage. It distinguishes them, for example, from counsellors and psychotherapists, who often use other kinds of utterances, such as offering interpretations ('*I think your symptoms are an expression of unresolved grief*'), using encouraging phrases ('*go on*', '*tell me more*') or simply reflecting back what the patient has just said. It is also helpful that patients in primary care settings expect to be asked questions and are generally prepared to give answers. In many ways, therefore, the surgery or community clinic is already set up for the process of narrative enquiry.

However, circular questions, as introduced in Chapter 2, are generally quite different from the traditional medical or nursing enquiry. The principal difference is that medical questioning is often aimed at narrowing down possibilities, whereas circular questioning is aimed at opening them up. This is not in order to have a longer encounter, but in order to use time in the most efficient way, by seeking exactly the words and contexts it is most important to pursue. All the questions that the nurse has asked qualify as circular questions, in at least two ways. First, they are all framed in direct response to the exact words used by the patient. Second, they all seek to explore the wider, interactive context for what the patient is saying about his experiences. Her questioning continues in the same vein.

> Nurse: I'm really sorry. What effects do you think that has had on you?
> Patient: It's made me pretty nervy that the same sort of thing is going to happen in my case.

The nurse in the above extract has, both literally and metaphorically, gone to the heart of the matter. She has defined exactly the task that is most likely to create a new story for the patient. It is a story in which he becomes less 'nervy' because he has the information to set his mind at rest.

In family therapy, many attempts have been made to codify the different kinds of circular question that can be asked. (Penn 1983; Tomm 1998). It is certainly helpful, at least for the beginner, to have a repertoire of possible questions to open up ideas of interaction and circularity, at least when acquiring the technique for the first time. One simple list, for example, includes the following (Launer 1999):

- Ranking questions (which is the most/least . . .)
- Speculative (what would happen if . . . ?)
- Relational (what effect would it have on you if someone in your family . . . ?)
- Contextualising (if you lived somewhere else, if you were younger/older, what difference would this make . . . ?)
- Introducing difference (what would need to happen . . . ?)
- Worst case (supposing nothing changed . . . ?)

There is also a particular kind of circular question that seems to help patients more than any other. This is the so-called 'reflexive' question (Tomm 1987b). Reflexive questions are ones that invite patients to consider familiar issues in unfamiliar contexts or from a new perspective. (The nurse in this case asks exactly such a question later, when she invites the patient to put himself in her shoes.) These are the questions that seem to 'stop patients in their tracks' in the most creative way. They are the ones most likely to nudge a story that is repetitive and stuck into one that is freer and more imaginative.

However, there are two important cautions that need to be given with any list of questions. The first is that it is a fallacy to believe that co-creating a good story depends on questioning alone. The technical purist who pursues an interrogation that is never punctuated with comments, advice, expressions of sympathy, humour or spontaneous thoughts is unlikely to make the human connections needed for a good story to emerge. Also, questions should never be formulaic and rigid: lists are meant as starting points only. The most important thing is for questions to convey an overall impression of circularity. This means taking every opportunity to indicate that stories are made up through dynamic conversations that can proceed in an infinite number of ways.

Although medical and circular questions are generally different, they do share some similarities as well. Some conventional medical questions also happen to fall into the category of circular questions. All those familiar litanies (*How long? Where? What makes it better? What makes it worse?*) can provide an easy entry into creating a much more broad-ranging narrative (*When was the worst time ever? What was your understanding of why it happened at that time? When do you get fears it might return as badly?*). This means that it is perfectly possible to track the patient's language closely, to follow feedback and still carry out the medical task. The nurse in this consultation demonstrates that it is possible to move between biomedical and narrative modes of inquiry – and to integrate safe biomedical questions, based on expert knowledge, into a narrative-based consulting style. (Further illustrations of circular questions appear at a number of points later in the book, especially in Chapter 6.)

It is of course impossible to learn any questioning technique from the written word alone. Circular questioning, like any other technique, can only be learned by constant trial and error. It is worth learning to avoid the questions that regularly seem to lead to a repetition of the same story or a deepening sense of inertia. By contrast, it is worth paying even more attention to the questions that appear to open up chinks of light in the narrative darkness. A sign of this can be a hopeful phrase such as: *'That's made me remember something . . .'* or *'There is one difference I wanted to mention'* or *'It's funny you should ask me that . . .'*.

Strategising

Clinicians in primary care bring to their work a repertoire of established strategies for consulting with patients. They employ some of these to meet the needs of the patients, for example attempting to solve their problems. They also devise strategies to meet their own needs, such as getting the patient out of the door on time. The strategies often have a complex history. They may come from training, or from textbooks on consulting technique, or as part of the collective lore of the profession. Often they have been refined by trial and error so that they have elements of both the personal and the professional in them. They may also include the use of standardised explanations or advice: for example, the repetitive phrases that GPs and practice nurses use to explain why there is no point in giving antibiotics for colds and flu.

Although strategising in a consultation is always necessary, practitioners vary in their awareness of them. Some people appear to go into a routine of giving advice or writing a prescription in most situations. They may be unaware that they are making particular choices about how to strategise, or that there are other choices available. By contrast, therapeutic strategising means developing the skill to notice how one has to make choices about how to proceed at almost any juncture in any consultation, and that these choices can often be shared with the patient. The nurse in the case vignette is doing this continually, and as we return to the consultation we find her doing it once more.

Nurse: Are there things we can do to help you find out, or prevent it happening?

Patient: I'd never really thought of that. It certainly wasn't why I came today.

Nurse: No, but we might be able to deal with the sore throat now and bring you back to check out your risks of heart disease.

Patient: To be honest, I'm not entirely sure I want to go into that. If it's in my genes, I'd rather not know.

The case for cultivating an awareness of one's strategies is similar to the case for becoming more conscious of the hypothesising process.

- It is more likely that one will notice the effect of helpful or unhelpful strategies on the patient.
- It is less likely that one will abuse the power of one's professional role by pursuing strategies that have little or no relevance for the patient.

Strategising can happen in relation to many aspects of the consultation. As the case example shows, it can be used to indicate constraints of time or resources. It can express itself in moves from silence to active involvement in the consultation. It can also take the form of deciding when to move out of linear questions and into circular ones, or vice versa. One form of strategising consists of deciding whether to try and nudge the narrative in a particular kind of direction. Nudging can be done hamfistedly (*'I want you out of the room so I am going to tell you that you'll definitely feel better in two days'*). But it can also be done experimentally, as it were, to see if the new narrative thread might be acceptable, and with a willingness to back off if it is not.

Sharing power

There are two dimensions to empowerment: empowering the patient and empowering the professional.

Empowerment of the patient is clearly at the heart of a narrative approach. Every technique is aimed at helping the patient to lead the narrative, and to share in the choices and dilemmas that have to be addressed. Empowerment is not just about sharing the final decision about what to do. It is about looking for opportunities at every moment in the consultation to hand over power. Nowhere is this more important than in the minute-to-minute conduct of the consultation itself.

Nurse: That's an interesting dilemma. If you were in my shoes now as the practice nurse, would you try and offer some screening tests like cholesterol, or would you back off?

Patient: That's an interesting question. I guess your job is to persuade people to have their cholesterol measured.

In some ways it is still very counter-cultural for practitioners to ask patients to make decisions in this way. It requires an ability to observe one's own role in an interaction and to comment on this freely to the patient. The nurse demonstrates it here by inviting the patient to imagine himself in her position. This skill calls for a certain level of sophistication and a degree of confidence. Yet once they have acquired it, practitioners seem to find this approach to decision sharing very liberating.

Usually the professional has more power than the patient. This is because professionals have expert knowledge and the power to permit or refuse access to a vast range of resources, including prescription medicines, hospital referral and state benefits. Professionals are often, though not always, representatives of a dominant cultural group in terms of gender, class or ethnicity. It is usually the professionals who, when the chips are down, can say how things should be organised and what the limits of negotiation are. For all these reasons, it is professionals who should be looking for opportunities throughout every consultation to share power, as the nurse does here, rather than to impose it.

At the same time, it is important to recognise that there are many ways in which health professionals can themselves lack power too. Many are severely constrained by their own working contexts, especially in such matters as the time available for consultation, the impoverished nature of their own support systems and the limited scale of the resources that may exist locally for onward referral. Within the health service, they may also see themselves as representatives of disadvantaged groups in society – for example, as female Afro-Caribbean nurses. Seen in this light, it is important to emphasise that there may be other situations, different from the one illustrated here, where it is quite appropriate to discuss the limitations of the work setting and of the clinician's authority within the system.

Reflection

One of the things that is perhaps most evident in the behaviour of the nurse in the illustration case in this chapter is that she is actively reflecting on everything she says, as she does again now.

> Nurse: [after some thought] No, my job is to offer it. Your job is to choose whether you want me to.
>
> Patient: I guess it would make sense for me to come back and get these things sorted out.

It is impossible to carry out conversations of the kind described here without making space for reflection. In formal family therapy, therapists use all kinds of aids to make sure they can do this. They have discussions with their teams before and after sessions, and often take mid-session breaks as well. The team may observe the session through a one-way screen or by video link (Tomm 1984). Or they may have a small group of colleagues in the room, breaking from time to time to hold a discussion with these colleagues that the patient can overhear – the so-called reflecting team (Andersen 1987). The idea of all these elaborate aids is so that the therapist can reflect on the content and process of the session, to develop a greater and more effective range of hypotheses, questions and strategies for the next stages of the work.

While all these techniques can and have been used to a very limited extent for research and training within primary care (Mayer *et al.* 1996), it would be absurd to suggest they might become established there as a routine. Yet, taken together, they represent an essential aspect of all narrative-based work: the need for adequate mental and emotional processing of the immensely complex information that can emerge from any interaction. The very scale and technological sophistication of the effort that therapists make to ensure this can happen draws attention to the almost total lack of support for the clinician in primary care who wants to reflect on what he or she is doing.

The stark contrast may be helpful, because it leads people in primary care to think about what is practicable as an aid to reflection in the context of very short consultations. This can lead them to adopt other measures, such as breaks in difficult consultations to exchange thoughts briefly with a colleague in the next room. It can also lead to a style of working that involves staging encounters over two or more consultations, rather than trying to compress them into one. And it can lead practices to examine their appointment systems to see if there is capacity for longer appointment slots in recognition of the complexity of much of the work. However, the most important type of reflection is undoubtedly what goes on inside the practitioner's head: a constant process of observation and monitoring that takes note of each intervention and its effect, and modulates the next intervention in response. This may involve short silences (as it does at this point in the nurse's consultation) but it may also show itself in a more carefully paced consultation that allows time for both parties to think about what they want to say, or a willingness to continue for a further episode.

Nurse: I'd certainly be happy to help you do that.
Patient: But in the meantime, what can you do about my sore throat?
Nurse: Mainly giving advice and reassurance. Gargling with salt water may help. And it'll probably go by itself in a few days.
Patient: Fine, I guess my main worry was about my heart, and if you're pretty sure it's not that ...

Finding a good new story

There is no point in learning or applying techniques unless they have a purpose. Within a narrative approach, the purpose of any technique must be to increase the chances of creating a good new story.

How do you know if the new story is a good one? All kinds of theoretical answers have been offered to this question. Most writers seem to agree that good stories are ones that are:

- coherent (Anderson and Goolishian 1992)
- aesthetically appealing (Keeney 1983)
- useful for the patient (Shapiro 1993; Amundson 1996).

Coherence is what distinguishes stories that have been clarified from ones that still contain inherent muddles or puzzles. Aesthetic appeal is something that, at first sight, may appear to belong to the world of the novel or art gallery than the clinic. Yet many practitioners will instinctively recognise that good consultations, and good stories, demonstrate a kind of internal harmony; they leave patients and practitioners with a definite sense of shape, clarity and closure. As a touchstone for a good story, however, usefulness is of greatest importance. If the story at the end of the consultation does not have efficacy for that particular patient, it has clearly failed. If it does, it has succeeded, as this one appears to have done.

Nurse:	Actually, I am.
Patient:	So when should I book an appointment to get the other stuff sorted?
Nurse:	Does two weeks sound OK?
Patient:	Two weeks sounds fine.

In primary care, the success or otherwise of the story may to some extent depend on circumstances and luck. For example, in the particular consultation illustrated here, the nurse will probably not know how good a story this is until a fortnight has passed. If the patient is admitted to hospital in the meantime with quinsy or (even worse) a heart attack, the story will not have been a good one. If he does not turn up to his next appointment and she never sees him again, she may never know if it was good.

However, in all likelihood, the patient will return having reflected on the conversation. He may well report that his own story has moved on in certain respects. He may have decided that he is now capable of facing his fears of serious illness by doing whatever investigations are necessary. Alternatively, he may report that he would prefer to live without a precise estimate of his risks and to enjoy life in a less medicalised state. Or he may come in with an entirely different story, but at least he now has a creative working relationship with the nurse in which old stories can be exchanged for new ones.

Suggested exercises

- Look back at a consultation. Try to recall the hypotheses you formed. Were these mainly medical or did they range into other areas? How did you test them? Were there any hypotheses that you tried out and then dropped? Are there any alternative ones you could have considered?

- Try to observe your own ways of strategising during a consultation. How far do you share these with the patient?
- After a surgery or clinic, consider the different resources for reflection that you used. What other resources could you have used?
- Choose one or two of the above techniques and consider how you might want to extend your use of them. Pick a consultation when you are not too busy and try doing so.
- Consider the three criteria for a 'good story' and add some of your own. Try to assess whether they fit some actual consultations, and if so what 'scores' are reached on each of them.

The consultation

Patient: I've got a sore throat.

Nurse: Tell me about it.

Patient: I'm surprised how painful an ordinary sore throat can be.

Nurse: I wonder why that is. Is it quite unusual for you to have this kind of thing?

Patient: It's not just that. I'm concerned the pain has lasted so long.

Nurse: That's not uncommon, but if it's your first it can be a bit of a shock. Are there any particular concerns you have about it?

Patient: Well, maybe I'm being a complete hypochondriac, but I've heard that heart trouble can make your throat hurt.

Nurse: Your symptoms sound quite different, but are there other things making you worry it's your heart?

Patient: Apart from my throat, nothing else is hurting.

Nurse: Is there any other reason you might worry about heart disease?

Patient: Yes, my father had a lot of heart trouble and he died from a heart attack last year. He was only 49.

Nurse: I'm really sorry. What effects do you think that has had on you?

Patient: It's made me pretty nervy that the same sort of thing is going to happen in my case.

Nurse: Are there things we can do here to help you find out, or prevent it happening?

Patient: I'd never really thought of that. It certainly wasn't why I came today.

Nurse: No, but we might be able to deal with the sore throat now and bring you back to check out your risks of heart disease.

Patient: To be honest, I'm not entirely sure I want to go into that. If it's in my genes, I'd rather not know.

Nurse: That's an interesting dilemma. If you were in my shoes now as the practice nurse, would you try and offer some screening tests like cholesterol, or would you back off?

Patient: That's an interesting question. I guess your job is to persuade people to have their cholesterol measured.

Nurse: [after some thought] No, my job is to offer it. Your job is to choose whether you want me to.

Patient: I guess it would make sense for me to come back and get these things sorted out.

Nurse: I'd certainly be happy to help you do that.

Patient: But in the meantime, what can you do about my sore throat?

Nurse: Mainly giving advice and reassurance. Gargling with salt water may help. And it'll probably go by itself in a few days.

Patient: Fine, I guess my main worry was about my heart, and if you're pretty sure it's not that . . .

Nurse: Actually, I am.

Patient: So when should I book an appointment to get the other stuff sorted?

Nurse: Does two weeks sound OK?

Patient: Two weeks sounds fine.

An extract from the sources

There seem to be some advantages for a therapist to ask mainly questions, especially in the early and middle parts of an interview. For instance, doing so tends to ensure a client-centred conversation. The perceptions, experiences, reactions, concerns, goals, plans and so on of the client are repeatedly called forth and take centre stage. If the therapist responds to the client's answers with further questions, the experience and beliefs of the therapist remain in a supportive role as the conversation unfolds. Thus, when the balance is in favour of questions over statements, the 'work' of the session naturally centres on the client, not on the therapist. Another advantage is that questions constitute a much stronger invitation for clients to become engaged in the conversation than do statements. The grammatical form of a sentence that poses a question arouses the social expectation for an answer. The cadence, tone and ensuing pause in the therapist's speech add to the expectation for a response. When the therapist also conveys a clear commitment to listen, and to hear the client's answers, the expectancy is strengthened even further. Thus, through questioning, clients are actively drawn into dialogue with the therapist . . .

A further advantage in therapists mainly asking questions and refraining from making statements, is that clients are thereby stimulated to think through their problems on their own. This fosters client autonomy and allows a greater sense of personal achievement . . . .

Karl Tomm (1988)

References

Amundson J (1996) Why pragmatics are probably enough for now. *Fam Proc.* **35**: 473–86.

Andersen T (1987) The reflecting team: dialogue and metadialogue. *Fam Proc.* **26**: 415–28.

Anderson H and Goolishian H (1992) The client is the expert: a not-knowing approach to therapy. In: S McNamee and K Gergen (eds) *Therapy as Social Construction.* Sage, London.

Keeney B (1983) *Aesthetics of Change.* Guilford, New York.

Launer J (1999) Teaching systemic general practice: a guide to conducting group exercises, III: developing interview skills. *Educ Gen Pract.* **10**: 72–5.

Mayer R, Graham H, Schuberth C, Launer J, Tomson D and Czauderna J (1996) Family systems ideas in the 10-minute consultation: using a reflecting partner or observing team in a surgery. *Br J Gen Pract.* **46**: 226–30.

Palazzoli Selvini M, Boscolo L, Cecchin G and Prata G (1980) Hypothesising-circularity-neutrality: three guidelines for the conductor of the session. *Fam Proc.* **19**: 3–12.

Penn P (1983) Circular questioning. *Fam Proc.* **21**: 267–80.

Shapiro J (1993) The use of narrative in the doctor-patient encounter. *Fam Sys Med.* **11**: 47–53.

Shawver L (2001) If Wittgenstein and Lyotard could talk with Jack and Jill: towards post modern family therapy. *J Fam Ther.* **23**: 232–52.

Tomm K (1984) One perspective on the Milan systemic approach: Part II. Description of session format, interviewing style and interventions. *J Marital Fam Ther.* **10**: 253–71.

Tomm K (1987a) Interventive interviewing: Part I. Strategizing as a fourth guideline for the therapist. *Fam Proc.* **26**: 3–13.

Tomm K (1987b) Interventive interviewing: Part II. Reflexive questioning as a means to enable self-healing. *Fam Proc.* **26**: 167–83.

Tomm K (1988) Interventive interviewing: Part III. Intending to ask lineal, circular, strategic or reflexive questions? *Fam Proc.* **27**: 1–15.

CHAPTER 4

Helping narratives to flow

'The quest is always for a more elaborated, all-embracing, spontaneous, individualised, flexible story that encompasses a greater range of experience.'
Jeremy Holmes (1998)

This chapter offers some specific suggestions regarding the kinds of consulting behaviour that may aid the development of new narratives. It also looks at ways of integrating a wide range of familiar activities in primary care using a narrative-based approach.

Key ideas in this chapter

- There are some straightforward ways of incorporating activities like physical examination, prescribing, health promotion and the application of scientific evidence into a narrative-based approach.
- It may be possible to adopt specific kinds of behaviour that invite more helpful and coherent narratives in primary care.

Points to consider

- How much do you find that 'conventional' professional tasks impede the flow of patients' narratives?
- What strategies do you have for incorporating these tasks into the consultation?
- How do you balance your needs as a professional to do certain tasks and the patient's needs to develop a better story?

The ideas presented here are a compendium of hints and tips that we have built up collaboratively with students. They are not meant as inflexible guidelines. A narrative-based approach is in many ways meant to counterbalance one based on consultation guidelines. Nevertheless, people who try out narrative ideas do notice patterns of speech and consulting behaviour that are particularly helpful. This chapter explores these, giving some suggested responses that we have evolved with students to 'frequently asked questions'. Not surprisingly, much of the guidance here converges with some of the recommendations for good practice that other primary care educators have made (Silverman *et al.* 1998).

Frequently asked questions: some hints and tips
How should I prepare for the consultation?

It is hard to set the scene for narrative-based consultation without a minimum of mental preparation, even if this only lasts half a minute. Many people trying to develop such an approach have adopted the habit of reading the notes or computer record before calling each patient, in order to recall 'the story so far'. This usually gives rise to some spontaneous hypotheses and questions forming in the practitioner's mind. It can be especially useful to try and give these hypotheses a definite shape rather than a vague one: for example, what are the possible or likely outcomes following the last episode of the story, and what might be useful questions to pursue?

Going to fetch the patient or family personally gives the opportunity for further possibilities to come to mind, perhaps based on body language or on the particular combination of family members who have turned up on this occasion. The quality of the reflective space the professional manages to set aside in advance, however brief, may determine the possibilities for new narratives to develop.

> One GP reported: 'In the past I never looked at the notes before calling someone through. I thought there just wasn't the time. However, I've now started doing it. Last week I saw a woman who lost her husband a year ago, and when I looked at her notes I realised it was the first anniversary of his death – the exact day. She was really touched that I was aware of this. It was extraordinary that I had noticed, and it transformed the consultation.'

How should I start the consultation?

From a narrative point of view, there is no reason to avoid one of the conventional questions, such as 'How can I help you?' Some people say nothing, and an expectant facial expression usually brings forth the patient's first statement.

We counsel against the use of formulations such as 'What's the problem?', since this already closes down some possibilities (for example, there may not be a problem or there may be several). Even when the practitioner is pretty sure what the consultation is about, it may still be worth checking out, for example by saying: '*Am I right in thinking you've come to have your blood pressure checked?*'

> Another GP told us: 'A man came in and said: "I've got four problems."
> I asked immediately: "Is there a fifth?" He looked surprised but said yes and
> he told me about it. It was the most important problem and we spent the
> whole consultation talking about it. He seemed to forget the other pro-
> blems. I'm not sure what made me take the risk and ask him something so
> bold. It may have been his body language, or just intuition.'

What about taking notes?

In order to signal an emphasis on oral narrative, it is helpful to keep note taking during the consultation to a minimum. As well as detracting from eye contact, taking notes lessens the amount of attentiveness available for the patient and the opportunity for reflection on the clinician's part. Clearly, there are situations when clinicians do need to jot some things down, such as blood pressure and peak flow readings, but it is possible to do this on a scrap of paper and transfer the details to the main written record or computer screen afterwards. To lessen distraction, it helps to have the computer screen switched off (or showing a neutral 'screen saver') during the consultation.

Some people say they cannot imagine keeping to time without taking notes in the consultation. However, most practitioners find that uninterrupted atten-tion makes things move along more quickly, so that there is enough time left over for making a record afterwards. In addition, writing the notes afterwards may make it possible to write a more concise and focused account of what has passed.

It can also be useful to include some brief information about the consultation process itself in the notes, particularly if this may point towards useful questions that can be raised at the next encounter with the patient.

> A GP explained: 'I often see a young man who is depressed and also rather
> isolated. He often tells me about how people have let him down: family,
> friends, social workers, the citizens advice bureau and so on. Last week he
> came in with another catalogue of disappointments. It occurred to me to
> ask him if he could think of any occasions recently when someone actually
> provided something he had asked for, and also whether he'd ever been able
> to influence anyone to do this. The question made him think. He couldn't
> recall anything then and there, but I suggested he should look out for this

until I see him in a couple of weeks. I've made a note of the suggestion so I can check next time if it's had any effect.'

How can I think of lots of good questions – particularly circular ones – to help narratives develop?

This is a very common question from people learning a narrative-based approach. It is tempting to offer a vast and comprehensive check list in response but, as explained in Chapter 3, this would be counter-productive. It could lead to highly stilted interviews, undertaken by rote instead of through following feedback. Nevertheless, a few principles appear to help people to develop a repertoire of good questions and a facility in crafting new ones.

- Pick up words or phrases that the patient has just said and use these as starting points for further enquiry.
- Focus on developing a general sense of process and circularity in the interview, rather than worrying about technical prowess.
- If a question doesn't yield useful information, don't repeat it. Ask a different one.
- Keep questions short. Don't add long explanations to each question. Ask one at a time, not a whole catalogue.
- If the patient answers a question you didn't ask, go with the flow!
- Over time, build up your own collection of effective questions – by trial and error, by observing others at work and by reading.

One of the most effective way of moving narratives forward is to ask questions that draw attention to the underlying values or beliefs that appear to be guiding people's behaviour. An example of this might be: '*Your husband seems to have a view that your disability is less than you believe. What do you think you might need to do in order to convince him otherwise?*' Although elaborate questions like this can seem unwieldy at first, they can yield very powerful results if well thought out and well timed.

How do you fit in physical examination?

Physical examinations can disrupt the narrative flow of an encounter. However, this can be lessened, by placing it within a narrative framework. This can be done by seeking permission, or by offering an explanation.

- *'Is it all right if I listen to your chest at this point?'* or
- *'I could get some useful information by checking the pulses in your feet. Is it OK if I do that?'*

Although such questions can seem rather precious at first, they are useful because they set a context for what the practitioner is doing. This enhances the sense of collaboration.

What about prescribing?

Many doctors and nurses confess that they often write prescriptions as part of a strategy for bringing the patient's story to a close. There are obviously better ways of integrating a prescription into the narrative. From a narrative point of view, offering a prescription is just a suggestion for taking the story in one particular direction and is therefore open to further discussion. There are many occasions when it makes sense for doctors to declare a strong opinion either way about the need for drug treatment, and they can still make this clear without foreclosing the narrative. However, the prescription needs to end up fitting the story, rather than the other way round. From a narrative perspective alone there is nothing intrinsically right or wrong about prescribing antibiotics for dubious minor respiratory conditions. What matters is whether or not the clinician has created a context for discussing this.

> A nurse practitioner explained: 'In the past I used to get into serious tussles with parents about antibiotics for kids with colds. What I tend to do now is say, "Look, the child specialists tell us not to give antibiotics for colds, but a lot of parents feel helpless if they don't have something to give." I explained this to a mother last week and she said: "That's the real problem. But if I know it isn't going to help, I'd rather not give it." '

How can diagnosis fit in with the narrative?

From a narrative point of view, a diagnosis is a form of story, albeit a highly respectable one that often commands a great deal of popularity. A diagnosis may be useful to the patient and have a great deal of meaning for them (because, for example, they already know someone who has asthma, or psoriasis, or whatever). It may also help them because it places them within a community of fellow sufferers from the same condition and gives them a common language to use with the professionals they encounter.

At the same time, there are all sorts of risks to diagnostic labels. First, they can be so familiar to professionals that it is easy to lose sight of how they can have different meanings – or none at all – to patients. They can also close down any further discussion of the patient's unique experience of their condition, or the beliefs and ideas that accompany that experience. For that reason, it can be useful to have a repertoire of questions that can hedge any diagnosis that is proffered. These include questions like:

- '*Have you heard the word "ringworm" before?*'
- '*What do you understand by "angina", and what would you like me to explain about it?*'
- '*Has anyone else called this "asthma"? Did you find that helpful?*'
- '*Do you know anyone else who's been told they have osteoarthritis? How has it affected them?*'
- '*Do you think of this as depression yourself?*'
- '*Do you know what doctors generally mean by a stroke?*'

The most important aspect of a diagnosis is that it has an inescapable effect on the narrative itself. The act of naming alters what is named and how it is experienced (von Schlippe 2001). Sometimes, giving a name to a condition makes it seem more manageable (e.g. '*Now I know it is only osteoarthritis I will stop worrying about it*'). At other times, it can make the condition seem more intractable (e.g. '*Well if it's osteoarthritis I'm stuck with it for life*'). For a diagnosis to be helpful, the positive effects on the narrative must outweigh the negative. It also needs to be the starting point for the next episode of the story rather than a form of foreclosure.

Is it possible to give advice within a narrative-based approach?

No one could possibly work in primary care without giving advice and information a great deal of the time. From the point of view of narrative, the crucial issue is whether this is given in response to how the story is already evolving or whether it hijacks the conversation. It is probably helpful to reframe every piece of advice as a suggestion, and therefore as part of a dialogue rather than a monologue. One way that this can be done is by packaging advice within a question like: '*What do you think would happen if you tried . . . ?*' or '*Something that people often seem to find useful in this situation is . . . Do you think that might work in your case?'* However, this technique will fail unless the practitioner is committed to paying attention to the answer – even if it is an entirely negative one – and picking up the narrative thread from that point.

There are inevitably occasions when clinicians have to give very strong advice. For example, a doctor who has just diagnosed peritonitis does not want to sound as if the recommendation for urgent hospital treatment is tentative or requires a long and reflective discussion. Yet even on these relatively unusual occasions, it is still possible to put very assertive advice in dialogic form: *'I am going to have to tell you something quite alarming . . . but then I want you to let me know your reaction.'*

How can you fit in health promotion?

Given the contemporary emphasis in primary care on heath promotion, disease prevention and chronic disease management, it would be unprofessional to dis-tract practitioners from attending to these. As discussed earlier in this chapter, the crucial issue is about doing this transparently. With each changing empha-sis in primary care culture, new activities can be presented as having unchal-lengeable moral authority. Patients may experience this as paternalistic and authoritarian (Armstrong 1995). It certainly enhances the patient's autonomy to be given information about this context rather than for it to be ignored or concealed. If, for instance, a cervical smear needs to be done because the prac-tice protocol says it should, or because there is a financial penalty for not doing so, it may help to declare this context. Patients can then decide how to respond to this from their own personal perspective.

> A practice nurse said: 'I hate all the things I have to do to patients these days. I feel it stops me being a proper nurse and turns me into a kind of civil servant. I was so exasperated last week that I said this to a patient. I was surprised by her reaction. She said she always appreciated it when I checked her blood pressure or checked her records for smears and so on – even when she hadn't asked me to. For her, it was a sign I was a really good nurse because I thought about her needs, even ones she didn't know about.'

How much should one disclose about oneself?

Among counsellors and therapists, it is generally considered wrong to have family photos on the wall or to talk about where one is going on holiday.

By contrast, primary care is much closer to the everyday social world. The doctor or nurse who withholds such information is likely to be seen as stand-offish or even forbidding. Most primary care professionals work in settings where many of their patients know about their family circumstances and even about their own medical histories. What seems essential is for clinicians to decide for themselves what they feel comfortable about sharing from their own stories. This means giving clear signals about their own need for privacy. It also means using one's own experience in a way that does not hijack the patients' own agendas or intrude on their necessary preoccupation with their own problems. The doctor or nurse who is known to have suffered from a major illness, for example, may preface any offer of a disclosure with a question such as *'Would it be helpful if I shared my own experience?'* The patient who does not wish to hear about this will probably ignore the question anyway.

> A dentist told this story: 'I was off sick last year for two months. All my patients knew about this obviously because they saw my locum, and they realised that I was quite seriously ill. When I first came back, I tried to avoid talking about it but it just didn't work. What I have found now is how to talk about it just enough, but not too much. People want to express sympathy and reassure themselves that I'm well enough to work. It creates a real bond with people who have been through it themselves. But there are also times when I have to move the conversation on, because otherwise it isn't clear which of us is the patient.'

How can I manage patients who bring multiple problems?

This can be seen as a shared problem for clinician and patient. Most patients are aware that a professional's time is limited and that the work needs to be focused. The key for managing this well, as the case in Chapter 1 shows, seems to be to strategise the consultation jointly with the patient, and to strategise early. This might involve, for example, checking out at the very beginning of the consultation whether more than one problem has to be addressed, and sharing the preliminary work of time management with the patient.

- *'Are these all part of the same problem, or do we need to go about them one by one?'* or
- *'Supposing we only had time today to deal with one of these, which is the most pressing?'*

Time and its limitations generally go unmentioned in consultations, but there is absolutely no reason why this should be so and many reasons to challenge this convention.

How can I deal with patients who bring inappropriate problems?

Another related problem is that of patients who bring problems that are more appropriate for other professionals or other agencies. They may have come to the surgery mainly because it is accessible and free, or because their understanding of complex institutional structures and professional boundaries is limited. Perhaps what they really need is a lawyer, a benefits adviser, a housing officer or their MP. Alternatively, they may want their doctor to intervene on their behalf in an area where this is most unlikely to have any effect. Often, such patients subscribe to a story of professionals being part of the social establishment and therefore possessing a great deal of influence and power. Conversely, practitioners themselves are more likely to have a narrative about their own work that emphasises lack of resources, poor or limited access to other agencies and powerlessness outside a fairly narrow set of professional connections. Somehow the gap between the two narratives needs to be bridged in a way that avoids confrontation.

Two strategies seem to be both realistic and respectful in this situation:

- listening to the patient's story of need and helplessness without too readily foreclosing it
- responding with an educational narrative concerning what other agencies can and should offer rather than what the doctor or nurse cannot. For many practitioners, this sometimes involves advising patients how to negotiate with an inflexible bureaucracy or an under-resourced agency, in order to ensure that their needs and rights are met.

A GP said: 'A black woman came to see me, desperate to get her daughter into the local grammar school – rather than one nearest her which has a terrible reputation. She wanted me to write a medical report saying her child had all sorts of special needs, but there really wasn't anything in her notes to justify this. In the end I managed to have a conversation with her that wasn't really about her daughter at all, but about racial discrimination and about how she felt she'd never had a chance herself educationally. I didn't write a report but I hope she felt able to take on the system better and work out a way of getting her girl into the school she wants.'

How can I get an observer perspective on the consultation?

When learning narrative techniques in learning groups – for example through role play – people often find it helpful to have an observer present. Fortunately, there are many ways to create an observer perspective for oneself without the benefit of a learning group. First, there is the observer in one's own head, who can be looking at the interactions in the room while simultaneously being a participant in them. You can invite family members in the room to offer their observations and become collaborators in the encounter. Most clinicians have some opportunity, at least on a limited basis, to arrange consultations with one of their colleagues sitting in.

The observer does not need to have any training. Simply having another pair of eyes and ears, another mind, and another voice to offer some comments can alter the encounter. Registrars, medical students, trainee nurses and others who are present in the workplace in a learning capacity can be used as independent observers. Although they may be unskilled in a formal sense, their innocence might lead them to notice things that are going on that experienced professionals might not notice because they are used to sorting life's complex experiences into convenient boxes with unseemly speed.

> A GP trainer told this story: 'I had a new registrar sitting in with me, quite an experienced woman who'd had time off to have children. After one consultation the registrar just said about a patient: "What a lovely face she's got!" I was completely astonished. This was a patient I've always felt very irritated with, and I don't find anything lovely about her at all. My registrar's reaction really made me think about this woman, and how we've got stuck with each other. After that I had a conversation with the registrar about all the things I could ask the woman next time, to try and get out of this.'

How can I run to time?

Most people who are trying out new narrative techniques report that they are held up in their consultations. This is no different from GP registrars who come out of hospital practice and find at first that they are overwhelmed by the complex needs that patients bring to primary care. In both cases, this is inevitable as part of the learning process, and practitioners need to make allowances for it. On the positive side, once people have acquired proficiency, they report that they are much more adept at keeping within time boundaries than they ever were previously. One reason may be that they become more confident about making time limitations explicit, and about sharing decisions about time management with patients. Also, they may no longer strive to achieve the impossible because they have a more realistic sense of the contexts that govern and constrain their work.

Many clinicians who have adopted a narrative-based approach realise how ridiculous it is to try and cram an almost limitless agenda of six or seven problems, opportunistic health screening, preventive advice and empathic counselling all into ten minutes. They then discover how to share the story of their constraints with patients, in a descriptive rather than confrontational manner, and collaborate in setting priorities, doing things in stages or thinking about other resources elsewhere.

How should I end the consultation?

If all goes well in the creation of a new story, an appropriate ending will become apparent to the participants rather than having to be imposed arbitrarily. However, in primary care there is often not enough time to address all the patient's needs. Although this may not be fair, it is unavoidable. There are ways of making this clear. It is perfectly acceptable to say: *'We need to wind up for today.'* With practice, it is easily possible to make such statements in an entirely friendly and non-confrontational way, although it is surprising how nervous and guilt-ridden doctors and nurses can be about doing so for the first time. An invitation to the patient to choose the interval of time before their next consultation can help to bring about a negotiated ending.

How can I help colleagues to understand a narrative approach?

Just as it is probably unhelpful for anyone to become known as a 'Balint doctor', or a nurse 'with a special interest in counselling and family work', it is not particularly useful to acquire the label of being 'narrative-based'. It is certainly a problem if practitioners believe they are becoming superb narrative practitioners while their colleagues think they have become maverick or incompetent.

Aggressive attempts at 'teaching it to everyone' are likely to destabilise working relationships, which may have functioned well because of a respect for difference. Such attempts can also imply that teaching should only be a one-way street – something that is rarely the case. A better outcome is probably to be regarded just as a better GP, nurse, health visitor, pharmacist or whatever, without anyone knowing or caring precisely why. Influence by example (including the example of learning from other people) may have a more benign and beneficial effect than narrative-based evangelism.

A related issue is how to work alongside practitioners who take an indifferent or even a hostile stance towards a narrative approach, including specialists who are sharing care of the same patient. In these cases it may be particularly important to work inconspicuously, for a number of reasons.

- Patients rarely benefit from ideological conflicts among their professional carers.
- Concrete and linear views of the world generally carry more weight than subtle and evolutionary ones, so the narrative practitioner is likely to lose out in any competition between the two.
- The essence of a narrative approach is respect for *all* viewpoints and stories, and it must therefore find ways of incorporating oppositional voices too.

A health visitor said: 'I have been seeing a young mother who is also attending the local psychiatrist, who has decided she is schizophrenic. I'm really not sure she is. She's been the victim of a lot of abuse and she's often a bit confused, but I don't find the diagnosis helpful. However, I'm trying to be very careful not to challenge the psychiatrist or undermine him. What I do is to discuss with the patient what effect it has on her to have this label, and how different people react to it.'

How can I balance narrative and evidence?

Evidence-based medicine has been one of the dominant ideas influencing doctors and other health service workers in recent years. However, it is an idea – one might say a kind of story – that often does not have an easy correspondence with the stories that are brought into the consulting room (Greenhalgh 1998). The following two case examples are designed to show how tensions between evidence and narrative can express themselves in primary care. They are presented in a more formal fashion than the other vignettes in the chapter. Each is followed by a commentary pointing towards ways in which the tension between evidence and narrative might be lessened.

Case study 1

Mrs M is a 45-year-old woman with raised blood pressure. Her cholesterol is also high and she is very overweight. Her mother died of a stroke at the age of 50. An ECG and echocardiogram show that she has an enlarged left ventricle. Her doctor has entered her various risk factors on to his surgery computer and this gives her nearly a 40 per cent risk of a serious cardio-vascular event in the next ten years.

Mrs M says that she is not surprised that her blood pressure is high as she has a lot of stress in her job as a hospital orderly. However, she believes the problem cannot be very serious because she does not suffer from head-aches in the way her mother always did. She says she will try and lose weight by cutting out bread and potatoes but she is not keen to take drugs because she is sure they will make her feel nauseated just as anti-biotics always do.

Commentary: It is conventional to look at the doctor's version in a case like this as the reality of the situation, and to think that the patient's account is full of ignorance, confused logic and denial. However, it may be more useful to look at these two versions of reality as parallel stories. The doctor has a narrative inside his head that has been influenced by his own past encounters and life experiences in the same way as Mrs M. If he tries to persuade her to adopt his entire narrative concerning her problem, he may be no more likely to succeed than if she tried to convert him to hers. If he wins a technical success and she takes the drugs, she may do so with a sense of enduring disempowerment or resentment.

An alternative approach would be for the doctor to explore what room there might be for convergence between the two narratives. Does Mrs M, for example, know of anyone who has taken medication for blood pressure without ill effects? Conversely, can he as a doctor remember anyone like Mrs M whom he really did help to lose weight and manage without medication? By thinking of this encounter as a problem of discordant narratives, he may open up the possibility of a new story that both he and Mrs M can subscribe to.

Case study 2

Mr and Mrs J are a couple whose son Jake, age 2, has severe atopic eczema. Jake's parents say they are frantic at their inability to stop Jake scratching, and also because of sleep deprivation.

Their nurse practitioner knows there is evidence that they should be giving Jake daily baths, using copious amounts of skin emollients, and topical steroids in limited quantities. When she proposes this, however, their response is one of despondency. They cannot imagine fitting the regime of meticulous skin care into their lives, especially as they also have a 4-year-old and a new baby. They have also heard awful things about steroids. They say they would like to see a specialist for allergy tests.

Commentary: The tension here between narrative and evidence may arise because the parents' original narrative was not in fact about Jake's eczema but about their own helplessness and exhaustion. The way to reach a convergence of stories might be for the nurse to set aside for a moment her own chosen evidence-based narrative of treating Jake's skin and to concentrate instead on their unmanageable feelings.

For example, she might offer Mr and Mrs J an alternative narrative that described eczema as 'the itching disease'. She might also reassure them that parental desperation with eczema is extremely common, and might be especially heightened for parents with two other under-fives. This might lessen their sense of ineffectiveness and give them a chance to open up a story about taking more control of Jake's condition. If this happens, they may be more likely to heed her advice – or she may be more likely to agree to a referral as something that the parents need in order to take their own story forward.

Suggested exercises

- Review a consultation and consider how 'conventional' medical activity such as diagnosis and advice were incorporated into the narrative. Were there other ways this might have been done? What would the possible effects have been?
- Consider the rules or habits you adopt as your 'consulting etiquette' (e.g. the way you summon patients, the position you sit, how you take notes etc.). How far do these impede or facilitate narrative development? How might you change them?

An extract from the sources

Conversation is nothing more and nothing less than the everyday, rough-and-tumble adaptational processes that enable us to live together on this planet. Moreover, conversations are not necessarily fragile events that require special nurturing ... Yet some [social] constructionists insist on defining 'dialogue' in pale and limiting terms, as if only polite discussion and an 'openness' to alternative viewpoints qualify. It is naïve and restrictive to believe that positive gains are usually accomplished through calm, rational deliberations or that only in an atmosphere of studied neutrality can clients make progress towards their goals . . .

[Social] constructionism does not necessitate running therapy sessions . . . consulting with team members, avoiding diagnoses, de-emphasising genetic explanations, refraining from making strong predictions or refusing to tell clients what they ought to do. Under certain circumstances each of these therapeutic preferences may prove defensible.

Jay Efran and Leslie Clarfield (1992)

References

Armstrong D (1995) The rise of surveillance medicine. *Soc Health Illn*. **17**: 393–404.

Efran JS and Clarfield LE (1992) Constructionist therapy: sense and nonsense. In: S McNamee and K Gergen (eds) *Therapy as Social Construction*. Sage, London.

Greenhalgh T (1998) Narrative based medicine in an evidence based world. In: T Greenhalgh and B Hurwitz (eds) *Narrative Based Medicine: dialogue and discourse in clinical practice*. BMJ Books, London.

Holmes J (1998) Narrative in psychotherapy. In: T Greenhalgh and B Hurwitz (eds) *Narrative Based Medicine: dialogue and discourse in clinical practice*. BMJ Books, London.

Silverman J, Kurtz S and Draper J (1998) *Skills for Communicating with Patients*. Radcliffe Medical Press, Oxford.

von Schlippe A (2001) Talking about asthma: the semantic environments of physical disease. *Fam Sys Health*. **19**: 251–62.

CHAPTER 5

Families

'It is worthwhile trying to look at a family not as a collection of individuals, but as a living and developing unit of interdependent members, sharing common internal and external conditions, and showing interactions, reflecting in their life history as witnessed by a family doctor.'
FJA Huygen (1982)

This chapter is about the family dimension in patients' narratives. The first part of the chapter looks at conversations about the family when there is only one patient in the room. The second part is about having conversations with two or more family members at the same time.

Key ideas in this chapter

- For most patients, families play a central part in how they understand and experience their problems. Enquiry into the family dimension of people's lives is an essential part of a narrative approach.
- There are specific techniques for bringing the family into patients' narratives, including circular questions and the use of geneograms.
- Taking geneograms is not a formidable exercise. It can be short, simple and highly effective. Practitioners can easily adopt it as a routine narrative tool.
- Primary care offers enormous scope for working with families, whether the problem is an individual one or a shared family one. Such work can be brief and integrated with everyday care.

Points to consider

- How far is your own way of working oriented around families rather than individuals?
- Do you use family trees and if so, how? If not, might you find them useful?

- What technical problems do you face when you have more than one individual in the room, and how do you usually deal with them?
- Do you have any reservations about extending the family dimension of your work? How might you address these?

Talking with individuals about their families

Family stories are nearly always present in the room, even if only one patient is there physically. Family members are present in the life stories that people carry inside their heads. They are also there in remembered conversations or imagined ones. Many consultations will have been rehearsed in advance with someone in the family. Most will soon become the subject of a story told to the family at home afterwards. Our stories, and our identities themselves, are quintessentially family ones.

As some of the case illustrations so far have shown, it is often possible to make sense of someone's problem only by enquiring into the family conversations that have previously taken place. Some of the most revealing questions in the narrative practitioner's repertoire include the following.

- *'Who at home is most worried about your problem?'*
- *'Was it your decision to come today or did someone else suggest it?'*
- *'Have you talked about this problem to anyone in your family? What did they make of it?'*

Equally, it is sometimes only possible to develop or consolidate a new story by finding out who else needs to be involved in the process.

- *'What would help to reassure your wife that this wasn't a serious illness?'*
- *'How do you think you might explain the diagnosis to family and friends?'*
- *'Who is going to need the most convincing that you're treating yourself properly?'*

There are, however, many consultations when it helps to go beyond such questions and to explore a fuller picture of people's family backgrounds. The rest of this section describes how to carry out that kind of exploration.

Exploring personal identity through family history

Few of us define ourselves by our medical histories. We generally see ourselves more as the children of our parents, or the parents of our children, or as siblings, spouses or partners. Moreover, illnesses often have a profound impact on the family (Altschuler 1997; Altschuler and Dale 1999). Almost everyone in primary care seems to recognise this as true, and yet many still feel inhibited about making a family enquiry as routine a part of their professional encounters as, say, questions about physical functions or smoking habits. In fact, a careful family enquiry is rarely an intrusion. It can be introduced with a question as simple as: *'Can I ask a bit about your family background?'* or *'Who's at home these days?'* To make it entirely clear that the motive is not one of looking for blame, it sometimes helps to add: *'I find it helps me to understand people more if I know who's around in their lives.'*

Asking questions about the family is a way of moving from the professional's perspective of the story to the patient's (Jenkins and Asen 1992). Asking about the family's wellbeing and their history is therefore a fundamental narrative-making intervention for nearly any consultation. However, it is particularly powerful in developing a new story when other, more conventional methods are proving unproductive. Tomson suggests that a family enquiry is particularly useful with the following: 'depression, somatisation, psychosomatic problems, consultations where the heart sinks, stuckness on either part, behavioural problems, dependency on drugs, alcohol or the doctor, relationship difficulties, failed treatment regimes, unusual health beliefs' (Tomson 1996).

The following case shows how well, and how economically, such an approach can sometimes work.

Case study: Ali A

A nurse said: 'I was struggling to make a connection with a young Kurdish man, Ali A. He was attending for a new patient health screen. He gave one-word answers to all my questions, even though his English seemed quite good. So I decided to stop filling in the computer template for a couple of minutes and asked him about his family instead. He told me that he had left his parents and five siblings behind in Iraq. I asked: "Are they all safe?" He suddenly became highly animated. I felt it transformed the quality of the consultation.'

Geneograms: the basic tool for creating family narratives

Most family therapists take family trees (or geneograms) as a routine. Many people in primary care are reluctant to do so. The main worry seems to be that they cannot possibly set down the whole family in the time available, so should not start it. This is similar to believing that you should never listen to anyone's heart in primary care because you cannot routinely carry out a full cardio-vascular assessment! The analogy works well, because GPs and primary care nurses are extremely good at making pragmatic decisions about how little they need to do in order to carry out any task. If the basic task of taking a geneogram is seen as establishing the most crucial elements of the patient's life story, only a very few questions may be needed to accomplish this effectively. The formal phrase 'taking a geneogram' should not deter practitioners from jotting down an improvised diagram in a few seconds on a piece of scrap paper, which can amount to exactly the same thing.

Case study: Harold B

A GP explained: 'A man of about 38, Harold B, was telling me about unaccountable feelings of sadness and failure. These had appeared fairly suddenly the previous month. Nothing in his circumstances seemed to account for this. Everything in his family and working life seemed to be going so well. His oldest child had just reached the age of ten. I asked him a few questions about his family. He told me that his own father had died just after his tenth birthday – the same age his son had just reached! He was stunned when he made the connection. He burst out with all kinds of ideas. He realised how scared he was of dying himself now. He also said he had no idea of how to be a parent to a child older than ten. It was a quite dramatic consultation.'

The amount and kind of information worth including in a geneogram will depend entirely on the time available and the purpose of the consultation. An example of a geneogram taken down during a consultation appears on page 69.

Trying out a new story

In one way, a geneogram just establishes the bare bones of the patient's life story. However, from a narrative point of view it is the creative act itself – the live construction of a geneogram between practitioner and patient – that is crucial. It not only creates intimacy, but brings about new understanding and indeed new stories about how the past came to influence and determine the present. Giving a coherent account of the past and how it came to influence current

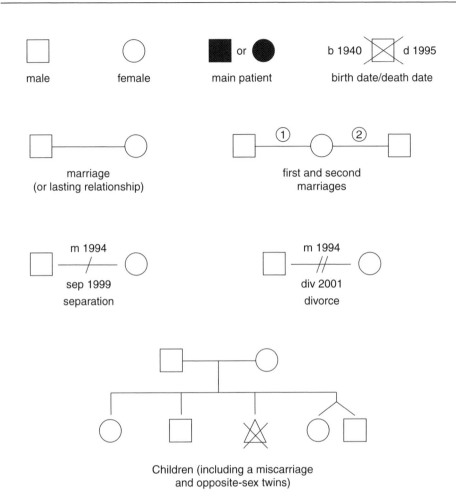

Figure 1   How to draw a geneogram.

difficulties can help people to identify what needs to be changed so that they can create a different story for themselves.

Case study: Karen N

Another GP told us: 'I have been seeing a woman called Karen N regularly while she has been going through a series of treatments for breast cancer. She has had a mastectomy, radiotherapy and chemotherapy. She keeps telling me about how she cannot stop being a 'coper'. She is always look-ing after everyone else including her husband and two daughters. She finds it impossible to take as much rest as she needs, even though her family seem fairly willing to help. I recently asked her a few questions about her family of origin. She was the eldest of five children. Her father was confined to bed for all of her teenage years because of spinal tuberculosis. She was effectively brought up as her mother's 'right hand'. She said it was hard to let go of control. We talked about this and she realised that her present family set up is far more supportive than the one she was brought up with. She is going to try to let others do more for her.'

Taking geneograms as a routine

Many GPs will think nothing of taking down elaborate past medical histories or health screening information for every new patient they see. Yet most would probably find the idea of taking geneograms systematically a rather intimidating one. This need not be the case. It probably takes much less time to elicit the basic family story for many people than it does to fill in the average computer template for a newly registered patient. And it may be far more effective in terms of the quantity and quality of information gathered (Tomson 1985).

Doing so leads to a more rounded understanding of the stories of many patients, especially those who are seen mainly in terms of their diseases or other superficial characteristics. It also makes it possible to see important connections between people who seemed unconnected – for example, married sisters with different surnames, or fathers and their married daughters – and to learn of significant members of the household who have never consulted or are registered elsewhere. It often produces important stories unexpectedly, especially when a doctor has become so familiarised with someone that he or she has developed an unvarying story about them. Perhaps because of this, routine taking of geneograms seems to produce a strongly positive effect on a doctor's perception of many patients. (It can also sometimes reveal a family history of disease or risk factors, such as diabetes or raised cholesterol, when this has been missed by other routine screening systems.)

Systematic taking of geneograms also helps to focus attention more on families with particularly troubling stories to tell. These include:

- early or repeated separations and disruptions in childhood
- the concurrence of two or more serious new diagnoses in the same household in a short space of time
- a family history of widespread major psychiatric disorder, from which the presenting patient might or might not have escaped
- childlessness and consequent isolation in the elderly, particularly useful in cases where the doctor has erroneously assumed that there was another generation of potential family carers

- existence of a previous marriage, and sometimes also of resulting children from whom the patient might now be estranged
- early parental death
- a history of immigration or emigration within the family
- a history of persecution and fleeing, with consequent separation from spouses, parents or children
- unconventional households (for example, elderly single brothers living together).

However, there can also be drawbacks to taking geneograms in an organised way. Like stamp collecting or train spotting, there is a risk that it can turn into an obsession that distracts practitioners from the primary purpose of enlarging their understanding. It requires discipline to recall that the point of taking geneograms in a clinical context is for their power to create new stories, not for the amassing of data in itself.

Case study: Irene M

A GP wrote: 'I saw an adolescent girl, Irene M, whose weight loss strongly suggested the early presentation of an eating disorder. I started her geneogram in the surgery. She became extremely enthusiastic about the idea and went home to construct an enormous six-generation geneogram on a sheet of unused wallpaper. She returned with her mother a fortnight later and proudly showed me the geneogram. We had a long discussion concerning the meaning of eating and food to the various generations of this family. Then her mother asked if I could test the daughter's urine. I did, and it showed three plusses of sugar and ketones.'

Conversations with the family present

People working in primary care have one tremendous advantage from the point of view of exploring family stories. Family members, in their twos and threes, attend surgeries in combinations of their own choosing as a matter of routine: as couples, as parents with young children or as children with old parents. These natural combinations do not need 'convening' – they just happen. There are many occasions when some sort of family conversation is therefore quite possible. All the practitioner needs to do is to notice these occasions and exploit the opportunities they provide for new narratives.

Everyone who enters the doctor's room for a consultation (or is present on a home visit) is in effect a participant in that consultation, even if their 'problem' is that they are concerned about the identified patient. The family member or neighbour who has apparently only been co-opted as a driver is sometimes the person who, with encouragement, will volunteer the most useful information. It may be worthwhile encouraging all patients, if they want to, to bring their partners, friends or neighbours into the consulting room rather than to leave them sitting in the waiting room because they have a mistaken belief that you might regard them as a nuisance. It may also be worthwhile to tell individual patients that you find it helpful to have somebody else from the family there to give another perspective. The response can be very surprising: a sister rather than a spouse, a neighbour of the same age rather than an adult child, someone from the church rather than from the family. Inevitably, some people will say no to the invitation, and this has to be respected.

Does such an approach lead to an overwhelming increase in workload? Often, the reverse is the case. This is usually because it is possible to elicit a clearer story as a result, or because there are more human resources for exploring a new one. Many experienced practitioners report that they find it easier and more productive to work with couples or larger numbers of people in the consultation than with individuals, because of the energy and the range of possibilities for new stories that this produces. With more than two patients in the room, there is a greater potential for asking questions about different perceptions, beliefs, theories or suggestions for treatment or for change.

However, it is also worth being cautious about actively inviting whole families to attend consultations together, unless one has a special interest in working this way. Although such invitations are standard practice in family therapy, they can seem intrusive in primary care or turn out to be unhelpful. Practical factors (small surgeries, too little time, inadequate materials for toddlers, nervousness about having enough skill) may spoil the encounter unless there is a lot of thought beforehand. It also goes against what people expect of their GP or practice nurse, so it may introduce an unnecessarily formal tone. Certainly, convening a whole family meeting is a very powerful intervention and should be offered with care: by a well-prepared clinician, to a suitable family, at the right time, and possibly with some kind of professional support like an observer or supervisor.

Involving the family in the conversation

Sometimes people come to primary care in twos or threes because there is 'a family problem', but usually this is not the case. They have come for other reasons, and they may want to express their views, but they do not want to go away feeling that they have a problem themselves or are part of the problem.

One way of including whoever is present without automatically casting them as patients is by the technique that family therapists describe as 'joining' a family. This means adopting the systematic habit of greeting everyone who arrives at the start of the consultation, finding out their identity and clarifying why they have come, unless it is perfectly obvious. By doing this, you can avoid discovering at the end of a consultation that the silent onlooker is deeply concerned about the patient and actually has a lot to say or ask. Making eye contact with everyone in the room at regular intervals is another way of indicating a willingness to hear everyone. It may encourage people to be forthcoming without any further prompting.

Although 'joining the family' sounds, and is, relatively simple – and many people in primary care do it instinctively – some doctors report that they have trouble doing it because of habits acquired in the past. These habits include focusing on the individual with the problem, while regarding everyone else as a kind of audience. However, once people have acquired the discipline of involving everyone in the conversation, they can be surprised by the people who speak up. This can include those with learning disabilities, toddlers, elderly people affected by Alzheimer's, and people whose English is poor and usually bring someone to speak on their behalf. Practitioners are also surprised by the variety of perspectives that can be present at the same time and the range of different stories that can come out as a result or turning individual consultations into joint ones. For example, relations are commonly bolder at speaking about the patient's unexpressed fears and may be more direct as their advocates when there is dissatisfaction.

Generally patients are very keen, and very relieved, when those accompanying them are brought into the orbit of the conversation, but sometimes they are not. They may even feel at risk of being upstaged. If this seems a possibility, it is important to ask permission before moving from a one-to-one dialogue into a wider conversation, for example by saying: '*Would you mind if I asked your daughter's view?*' or '*I'd find it helpful to hear what your wife has noticed. May I ask her?*' Such strategies make it possible to hear other descriptions of the problem and other suggestions for dealing with it. They also make it possible to help with a variety of different stories at the same time, for example the story of the worried relative along with the patient's story.

Case study: Eric R

A GP gave this account: 'Eric R and his mother have been registered with me for the past nine years following the retirement of their previous GP. The mother (now 79) has always been a frequent attender and has had cancer of the colon, asthma and osteoarthritis. The son (now 49) has asthma and has not worked since being made redundant from his job as a shop assistant a few years ago. They live together in a large house and have always seemed to have a close and protective relationship. They had a cat they adored, who died recently. A few months ago the son came to see me complaining of episodes of "spasms" in his throat, which caused difficulty in breathing, speaking and swallowing. He described the sensation as feeling as if someone had their hands round his throat. After these his voice was hoarse for several days. He had a long history of asthma but these symptoms were different.

'I referred him for an ENT opinion and all was found to be normal, including a barium swallow. I also referred him to see a speech therapist to learn relaxation techniques. The spasms continued and got worse. When I questioned him, he said he wasn't depressed or worried about anything. On a home visit the mother expressed concern about these symptoms as similar symptoms in the son's early twenties had resulted in several years of dependency on Valium. I felt I needed to know more about their life, so I listened while the mother talked. She told me how when the patient was five, his father came home after being in prison for several years. Eric had no previous memories of him. The next day they went out and the father became angry with the child while carrying him, as he would not sit the way he wanted him to. He shook the boy violently, and he was terrified and unable to breathe. The mother dates the start of his asthma from that moment.

'From the way she told this story it was obvious it had been told many times over the years and was a very significant family story to them. The son was diagnosed as having "severe nervous asthma" and was taken to see many doctors, both NHS and private, during his childhood. The father was frequently violent towards the mother but it was not until about ten years later, after he had broken her collarbone, that he left. The mother told everyone this was for financial reasons. It is striking how much effect this man, who they have not seen for many years and is probably dead, still has on their lives.

'On my next home visit I asked the mother some questions about the son's illness. I asked her what she thought his symptoms were caused by. She said she thought he had been depressed since the death of the cat a few months ago. The son accepted this idea. He had always denied being worried about his mother's health, so I asked the mother if she thought Eric worried about her. She replied that he did, but it was not necessary, and she had told him not to worry. I said that maybe it was unrealistic for him not to worry given the mother's health problems and maybe he should be allowed to worry. I also suggested that sometimes it was as difficult to watch someone being ill as to be ill oneself.

'I subsequently saw Eric on his own about his depression. I started him on antidepressants but he discontinued these due to side effects. However, over the next few weeks the throat symptoms resolved and he no longer seems depressed. The mother also seems happier, with fewer physical symptoms. My hypothesis was that the death of the cat reminded him that one day his mother will die and he will have to cope with life on his own. I think he is a very lonely person and I guess he may have sexual difficulties but I think this is probably as far as I should go in my enquiries, at least for the moment.'

Conversations with children

One dimension of family conversations requires specific attention. Children are present in a great proportion of primary care consultations but often no one actually speaks to them directly. GPs get no special training in how to engage children in conversations. Unless they have children themselves, they may lack confidence in doing so. Although they may know quite a lot about the development of things like motor skills, GPs may have little idea of the appropriate language and cognitive ability to expect of a child at any particular age. In addition, because the emphasis of medical training is so often on the objective diagnosis rather than the narrative encounter, many GPs may assume that it is enough to talk to parents *about* their children's experiences rather than to find out about these from the children themselves.

Fortunately, children are good teachers. Unlike adults, they will indicate that they have not understood a question by shrugging or looking blank rather than confabulating. This kind of feedback, although it seems rather brutal at first, is a good way of learning whether questions make sense or not. Most children, especially young ones, tolerate fewer questions than adults. On the other hand, making it a principle to ask questions of children in every consultation when they are present (even if the identified patient in the consultation is a parent) will prevent them being bored and unruly. Any child in the room with any level of verbal ability is a patient in his or her own right – and of course one can still communicate with pre-verbal children in other ways.

From a narrative point of view, the child too has a story to tell. It may be a naive story, but it may be all the more honest, vivid and telling because of that. It may contain important information, perhaps by its very contrast from the parent's account. If a clinician is confident and fluent in engaging children in conversation, and has taken the trouble to cultivate this skill, it will provide a good model for parents who want to develop this ability in themselves in order to give their children a clearer voice. Direct conversations with children can also be therapeutic for the children themselves, particularly if they feel as if they have had a chance to put their symptoms and worries into their own words, and if their anxieties can be allayed by face-to-face reassurance and explanations so that they can take away a better story than the one brought into the surgery (Dowling 1993).

Conversations about family problems

Families do not speak with one voice. They have many. On most occasions in primary care, these voices support or complement each other, but there are also times when they are in discord. This may be apparent from the beginning of the consultation, because they have intentionally come to discuss a relationship problem. On other occasions, the discord becomes apparent as disagreements emerge during the conversation itself. The initial story may have been about something like a medical problem, or depression, or a child's behaviour, but it then turns it into something else: an explicit family problem.

In dealing with family problems, some of the 'six Cs' concepts presented in Chapter 2 can be particularly helpful. An attitude of *curiosity* conveys that there is no 'right' or 'wrong' version of the story, and that the role of the doctor or nurse is not to adjudicate or choose among competing versions. This in turn indicates to the family that the consultation is a safe space for expressing differences and for exploring whether an agreed new narrative is possible.

Another mainstay of conversations with families is the use of *circularity*. Using circularity in this context involves several related techniques:

- allowing everyone an opportunity to speak, by inviting all their views and moving between them as equitably as possible
- indicating a belief that everyone has a continuous effect on everyone else, so that it is unproductive to try and determine 'who started it'
- following a mode of 'circular questioning' that invites people to move away from blaming and towards observing reciprocal effects and patterns.

One of the most helpful aspects of circularity is that it transmits the idea that there may not be a single solution to the family's difficulties, but at least there is an evolving conversation and therefore the possibility of changing the story. Even if the new story does not emerge in the consultation itself, the conversation has provided a model for how old stories become unglued and new stories are created.

Case study: Leo and Briony

A GP reported: 'This case involves a couple, Leo and Briony, both in their early twenties. He is Swedish and does computer work, she is from Wales and is a graphic designer. Leo came to see me saying he was glad I was a lady doctor and could he discuss his girlfriend's problem with me. He explained that it was a sexual matter and that he found it easier to talk to a woman about it. The problem was that his girlfriend of two years standing was no longer interested in sex with him, and for the last nine months would push him away and burst into tears. He talked openly about his worries about this – whether it could be a physical problem of hers or whether it might be all his fault – caused by him being unfaithful one year ago.

'I was curious that he was presenting "her" problem – he explained that she could not make this appointment. I asked him what his girlfriend would say was wrong if she were there. He said "she just says she doesn't know but she is very worried that she will lose me". We discussed his worries that she was upset with him and his frustration that this problem was persisting despite his sympathetic attitude. I suggested they return as a couple for a consultation with me with a view to possible referral for psychosexual counselling. He said they were not interested in a referral but would like to come back and see me anyway.

'Leo returned together with Briony. They sat close to each other holding hands. Briony said that her worst fear was the end of the relationship – they were each other's first sexual partners, and until he had been unfaithful, their only ones. He explained it had only been a one night stand, and that he had immediately telephoned Briony, who was visiting her parents in Wales, to tell her and apologise. I asked about her reaction – she had been devastated and nearly decided not to come back from Wales, but he called so often that she came back to rejoin him. Their sexual relationship initially continued as normal and then the problems began. I asked how she reacted at the time. They agreed she had been very angry initially but expressed it very calmly, which was usual for her. I asked her if she was still angry or upset about his unfaithfulness, and she said yes, she thought of it all the time. Leo then burst out in frustration "I've told you I'll never do it again and I'm sorry, what else can I do?" The couple seemed stuck in this painful state, but terrified of separating. I shared these thoughts with them.

'I was not sure if the discussion had any effect. However, the following month Briony came alone to talk about contraception, and she mentioned the difficulty she had had in expressing anger. She said that on the whole things were improving for them.'

GPs and nurses vary a great deal in how keen they are to tackle couple or family problems of this level of sensitivity in their everyday work. Some have been attracted to their jobs, and to further training, precisely because that is one of their interests. Others feel that they cannot offer the time or the skills to do this kind of work – and yet they recognise that it comes to them willy-nilly. Many families will not seek the help of any other agency, nor accept an onward refer-ral. For better or worse, primary care is 'de facto' the part of the health service where most actual family therapy happens. Brief work of the kind the GP did with Leo and Briony may achieve more than many practitioners might expect, and certainly more than a referral to another agency that the family does not wish to attend. While staying within the limits of their own interviewing skills and confidence, most practitioners seem to find it possible to extend their experi-ence of such work, and then find it unexpectedly gratifying. Those who go on to acquire some degree of training in this work generally report that it becomes a cornerstone in their way of practising.

Suggested exercises

- In a series of consultations, ask for some basic information about: 'Who's at home?' What difference does this make to the rest of those consultations?
- Choose one consultation when you are not too busy and where it seems appropriate to write down a more detailed geneogram. What light does it shed on the problem and what effect does it have on the story?
- Select two or three other ideas from this chapter (for example 'joining', asking children's views, asking questions of each family member in turn). How well does this fit with your normal practice? What effect does it have?
- Start to experiment with circular questions. Which ones seem to work and which do not?

An extract from the sources

The Canadian therapist Karl Tomm gives the following imaginary exam-ple of the difference between asking linear, circular and reflexive questions when interviewing a family. His suggestions are meant to demonstrate these forms of questioning, not to suggest that a real-life interview could or should proceed exactly along these lines.

Linear questioning
Interviewer: What problems brought you in to see me today?
Wife: It's mainly depression.
Interviewer: Who gets depressed?
Wife: My husband.
Interviewer: What gets you so depressed?
Husband: I don't know.

Interviewer:	Are you having difficulty sleeping?
Husband:	No.
Interviewer:	Have you lost or gained any weight?
Husband:	No.
Interviewer:	Do you have any other symptoms?
Husband:	No.
Interviewer:	Any illnesses lately?
Husband:	No.
Interviewer:	Do you have a lot of morbid thoughts?
Husband:	No.
Interviewer:	Are you down on yourself about something?
Husband:	No.
Interviewer:	There must be something troubling you. What could it be?
Husband:	I really don't know.
Interviewer:	Why do you think your husband gets depressed?
Wife:	I don't know either, he is just not motivated. He lies in bed all the time.
Interviewer:	How long has he been depressed?
Wife:	Three months. He has hardly been out of bed in three months.
Interviewer:	Did something happen that started it all?
Wife:	I can't remember anything in particular.
Interviewer:	Does anyone try to get him up?
Wife:	Not really.
Interviewer:	Why not?
Wife:	Well I get fed up after a while.
Interviewer:	Do you find yourself getting frustrated a lot?
Wife:	Quite a bit.
Interviewer:	How long have you been so frustrated?

Circular questioning

Interviewer:	How is that we find ourselves together today?
Wife:	I called because I am worried about my husband's depression.
Interviewer:	Who else worries?
Wife:	The kids.
Interviewer:	Who do you think worries the most?
Husband:	She does.
Interviewer:	Who do you imagine worries the least?
Husband:	I guess I do.
Interviewer:	What does she do when she worries?
Husband:	She complains a lot, mainly about money and bills.

Interviewer:	What do you do when she shows you that she is worrying?
Husband:	I don't bother her, just keep to myself.
Interviewer:	Who sees your wife worrying the most?
Husband:	The kids. They talk about it a lot.
Interviewer:	Do your kids agree?
Children:	Yes.
Interviewer:	What does your father usually do when you and your mother talk?
Child:	He usually goes to bed.
Interviewer:	And when your father goes to bed what does your mother do?
Child:	She just gets more worried.

Reflexive questions

Interviewer:	If you were to share with him how worried you were and how it was getting you down, what do you imagine he might think or do?
Wife:	I'm not sure.
Interviewer:	Let's imagine there was something that he was resentful about, but didn't want to tell you for fear of hurting your feelings, how could you convince him that you were strong enough to take it?
Wife:	Well, I'd just have to tell him I guess.

He writes: 'As the therapist asks questions to identify patterns ... family members who are listening to the answers make their own connections as well. Thus, they may be able to become aware of the circularity in their own interaction patterns. With this increased awareness they may be 'liberated' from the limitations of their prior lineal views and subsequently be able to approach their difficulties from a fresh perspective ... Questions are reflexive in that they are formulated to trigger family members to reflect upon the implications of their current perceptions and actions and to consider new options.'

Karl Tomm (1988)

References

Altschuler J (1997) *Working with Chronic Illness and Disability*. With contributions from Barbara Dale and John Byng-Hall. Macmillan, Basingstoke.

Altschuler J and Dale B (1999) On being an ill parent. *Clin Child Psychol Psychiatry.* **4**: 23–37.

Dowling E (1993) Are family therapists listening to the young? A psychological perspective. *J Fam Ther.* **15**: 403–11.

Huygen FJA (1982) *Family Medicine: the medical life history of families.* Brunner/Mazel, New York.

Jenkins H and Asen K (1992) Family therapy without the family: a framework for systemic practice. *J Fam Ther.* **14**: 1–14.

Tomm K (1988) Interventive interviewing: part III. Intending to ask lineal, circular, strategic, or reflexive questions? *Fam Proc.* **27**: 1–15.

Tomson D (1996) Constructing geneograms with patients and their families. *Context (Suppl: Thinking Families).* **Spring**: 6–7.

Tomson P (1985) Geneograms in general practice. *J Roy Soc Med (Suppl 1).* **78**: 34–9.

CHAPTER 6

Mental health

'The kinds of suffering that drive us mad are the kinds we say have no point.'
S Hauerwas (1993)

This chapter focuses mainly on problems that are usually described as 'mental health' problems.

Key ideas in this chapter

- Narrative ideas may provide a particularly useful framework for working with problems in the area of mental health.
- Narrative is not necessarily an alternative to conventional psychiatric diagnosis and treatment but can be integrated with this.
- By working with narratives, practitioners in primary care may be able to carry out a wide range of therapeutic work, including family work and crisis intervention, that is hard to offer in any other setting.

Points to consider

- In what ways might you find a narrative-based approach useful in handling the difficulties of dealing with people regarded as having mental problems?
- What are the risks of using such an approach and how can these be overcome?

A narrative approach to mental health

Many people in both primary care and psychiatry have reservations about current medical ways of thinking about mental health problems (Shepherd *et al.*

1986; Launer 1998; Bracken and Thomas 2001). They are concerned that labels including 'depression' or 'post-traumatic stress disorder' can pathologise many people who are simply grappling with adverse life experiences (Gremillion 1992; Cooksey and Brown 1998; Heath 1999; Middleton and Shaw 2000; Summerfield 2001). They also feel that such labels offer a poor fit with the complex and ambiguous ways in which people present to primary care (Armstrong 1996).

By contrast, an approach to mental health that is based on stories looks for accounts that have meaning for the patient, rather than labels that will satisfy the specialist. It tries to find a story to fit the uniqueness of what each patient is going through, while leaving open the possibility that conventional labels such as 'depression' might be useful in many instances. This is not an evasion of responsibility. It is a recognition that what matters is whether the words make sense to the patient, not whether the patient can be persuaded to accept a certain official designation.

Depression

Conventionally, doctors are trained to 'detect depression' by asking specific questions about the patient's experience – for example, early morning waking, weight loss and suicidal thoughts. Such questions certainly establish whether the patient's description measures up to the agreed professional notion of depression. That in itself may be useful for all sorts of reasons. It may help some patients who want to try and locate their experiences along the spectrum of other people's experiences, or who find it useful to have a name for what they are going through. It may also reassure doctors who want to make sure they are not forgetting to enquire about important indicators of personal risk. However, there are obvious problems too. A diagnosis can in itself be a form of pathologising or of amplifying and prolonging the problem. Also, by defining and concretising people's symptoms in this way, professionals may be distracted from meeting the patient's wider needs: to make fuller sense of their experiences and to explore their own preferred options for change.

An alternative, narrative framework for talking with people who appear to be depressed involves offering them the label of depression without insisting that it has to be relevant or useful. There are questions like:

- *'Would you describe what you are going through as depression?'* or
- *'Some doctors would give the name "depression" to what you are describing – would you find that useful in your own case?'*

Such questioning offers patients the landmark of a diagnosis if that is what they wish, without closing down dialogue or stigmatising them if it is not how they view their problems. Either way, it does not presuppose a particular form of treatment, since it leaves open the option of saying at a later stage in the consultation:

- *'Was it ever in your mind to try antidepressant pills for a while?'* or
- *'Would it be helpful for us to think about medication as one way of addressing your problems?'*

The point of such questioning strategies is to keep alive a sense of negotiability about symptoms, choices and the way forward. It also maintains the doctor's usefulness in the many instances where patients do not want to conceptualise their experiences simply in the way that the medical profession finds most convenient. It leaves open the possibility of alternative approaches, such as looking at the patient's geneogram or suggesting that a spouse or close relative might come along in order to give a wider understanding of what is going on. Most importantly, it lets patients choose the kinds of ways they want to define their story. That certainly includes the medical or psychiatric ways of conceptualising the world, and many patients are comfortable in choosing that way for themselves. However, a narrative approach is one that does not summarily close down other ways of understanding personal turmoil and distress.

At the same time, it is important to acknowledge the common-sense limits to a narrative approach of this kind. Faced with a patient with incapacitating or life-threatening patterns of thought and behaviour, it can be dangerous to pursue questions like this. However, the (rare) occurrence of extreme risks in primary care too often seems to constrain professionals from taking a more liberating approach in the generality of cases. Very often, it is possible to give permission to patients to take a more biographical approach to their experiences and to discuss their symptoms at the same time as addressing issues from their work, home life and family background. This can lead to the discovery of a middle ground where no one is minimising the degree of their suffering, nor are their problems being reduced to a single-word definition.

Case study: Meryem H

A GP told this story: 'Meryem H is about 50. She used to consult almost every week with symptoms of depression and tiredness. I always used to get bogged down with her. She has had four children, a boy of 19 who had left home three months ago to live by himself, another who would have been 21 but died in a swimming accident three years ago at the age of 18, and two girls in their mid-teens who were still living at home. She has divorced her husband. On the previous consultation she had come for a repeat prescription and had said how tired she felt. The latest antidepressants I had given her were no use.

'I realised I did not know her very well apart from the bare bones of her story and I wanted to start from scratch. I decided to offer her a long appointment for the following week to try and get to know her better.

'When she came back, she told me she has been increasingly depressed since the death of her oldest son. She talked about the guilt she felt if she did anything which might be construed as enjoying herself, so that she spent most of her time lying in bed blaming herself for past events, crying and visiting her son's grave. She was aware that her other children wanted her to do things like going shopping with her daughters. She felt unable to do this because she thought of her dead son all the time and she would end up crying if she went out with her other children. This made her feel guilty and she knew that they felt resentful of the dead brother who appeared to be her favourite child.

'She also felt guilty because she had known for many years that her marriage was not working. She feels that if she had split up with her husband years before then perhaps her son would not have died. As her other son approached the age at which his brother had died she was worried that something might happen to him too. She had tried to stop him moving away from home, and when he came round for meals now she would often cry and her son would hug her.

'I felt that it was very important to acknowledge the sadness of her story. I pointed out to her that she had managed to continue to be a good mother to her children and that they obviously wanted to spend time in her company even though one had left home. She was visibly moved by this statement. Her whole body language changed. She sat up and leaned forward in her chair to hear what was next. I took the risk of being quite directive and suggesting that she set aside a period of time each week for each of her children and devote that time to them individually to doing whatever each of them wished to do in that time.

'I now see her at intervals of three or four weeks to see how she is getting on with this. The approach seems to have worked. She does sometimes talk about her depression but far less. Mainly we just talk about her life, which now seems to be going somewhere, though slowly.'

Psychosis

People who experience psychotic thinking bring unusual and peculiar stories to the consultation. From the point of view of taking a narrative-based approach, there are probably two kinds of risk that can arise when dealing with their stories. One kind of risk is to discount everything the patient says as a mad story and therefore not worthy of any exploration. This effectively deprives them of the sort of conversation that takes place with every other patient, and is clearly unjust. Doctors nowadays are seeing it as increasingly important to provide good technical medical care to people who have been given the diagnosis of schizophrenia or paranoia; it may be equally important to see that they are also not excluded from normal and respectful discourse. Such exclusion only adds to their isolation and marginalisation.

The other kind of risk, however, is to be drawn into apparently delusional ideas to the point that one sees them as an equal reality to one's own. There are indeed practitioners who have taken this view within the worlds of psychiatry and of family therapy (Anderson and Goolishian 1992). However, there are probably two good reasons for not going to this extreme in the primary care setting:

- primary care clinicians work within professional networks where such a relativistic approach would still generally be seen as unethical and destructive
- it might prevent practitioners from noticing serious risk.

In practice, it does seem possible to hold conversations with psychotic patients that hover on the razor's edge, as it were. This means accepting their language in the context of the conversation, while not letting go of one's perception of them as disturbed, distressed and in need of protection. For example, it may be better to use the words: *'How long have people in the street been talking about you?'* rather than *'How long have you been thinking that people are talking about you?'* Such an approach has the advantage that one can enter the linguistic world of the patient without surrendering a hold on one's own more orthodox story about reality. Working in this way, on the borderline between rejection of the story and collusion with it, appears to enhance trust and to increase the possibility of having thoughtful conversations about things like medication.

Case study: Ben T

A practice nurse said: 'I see a schizophrenic man called Ben T regularly. He won't go to the mental health nurse, but he agrees to have his injections from me because he trusts me more. He always talks about people on "Death Row" in America. He says he writes them letters but I don't know how far that is true. Sometimes he cries when he talks about them. I think in a way he is talking about his own suffering but I don't think he would understand if I confronted him with this. Instead, I usually tell him that I regard his concern as a sign of how sensitive he is. We talk about the Death Row prisoners a lot and in a sense I suppose I am using it as a metaphor for him, but I don't think that really matters.'

Frequent consulters and 'heartsink patients'

Patients who make their own doctor's heart sink can often leave other doctors' hearts quite unaffected (Mathers *et al.* 1995). It might therefore be more appropriate to talk of heartsink interactions (Wright and Morgan 1990; Salinsky and Sackin 2001). It is worth speculating how doctors might alter their view of the matter by also considering which patients and families have the opposite effect: we call these 'heartleap patients'.

In the case of any heartsink interaction it can help to consider the following questions.

- What purpose does the stuckness serve? Are there reasons why a fixed story may be preferable to asking new questions, or to exploring alternative accounts of what is going on?
- What are the patient's contexts that are being ignored? Does the stuck story acquire meaning, and perhaps some negotiability, if more is known about the patient's geneogram, current household or working circumstances?
- Does the patient feel as stuck as the practitioner, or is there something comforting in the very repetitiveness of the story?
- Does the professional's inability to ask any new questions reflect the limitations of the working context (e.g. if I ask this question and she gives that answer, I still don't have anywhere I can send her)?
- What questions could the doctor ask that might challenge patients to describe their experiences in a different way? What questions might revive the doctor's curiosity and help them to see the patient not as annoying and burdensome but as someone unique, interesting and worthy of compassion?

Questions that seem useful in these kinds of interactions are often very broad ones, and also simple:

- *'What's the best thing going on in your life at the moment?'*
- *'Are there things in your life that you've never told me about that you think might help me to understand you better?'*
- *'I'm curious to know what keeps you coming back to doctors and having faith in them when they often don't seem to make anything better for you.'*
- *'I wanted to ask you how you view our consultations, and if you get anything out of them?'*

It would be idealistic to say that questions like these always turn repetitive interactions into sparklingly refreshing ones, but they do often yield surprising results, especially revelations from the patients that they have derived support and benefit from consultations that the doctor has felt were going nowhere. An equally common outcome is for the doctor or nurse to say: '*Until I'd asked that question and got an answer, I never really understood the patient. Now I feel I do.*' Inevitably, some interactions do continue like stuck recordings, in spite of the doctor's most imaginative efforts – but trying and failing to elicit a new story still makes the practitioner feel better than never having tried. It may also uncover the fact that frequent consultations about stuck problems are the 'least worst' option for the patient: they may be preferable, for example, to complete isolation or to suicide.

Perhaps the most impressive analysis ever written about a family of frequent consulters appears in a paper by Dowrick with the appealing title 'Why do the O'Sheas consult so often?' Dowrick shows how he and his GP colleagues attempted to unfreeze work with a family of frequent consulters bringing complex needs to the surgery. He and his team used a variety of tools to approach their work, including hypothesis generation, hypothesis testing and strategising. However, the core database for the work was a combination of the family geneogram coupled with information about the consultation rates of the various members. One striking correlation that emerged from this was between consulting behaviour and the loss of significant people – including doctors in the practice who retired (Dowrick 1992).

Somatisation and 'grey area' conditions like ME

There is an extensive literature about somatisation in primary care, with guidance about specific ways of addressing it. Much of the literature addresses ways in which patients might be influenced to talk about psychosocial issues in their lives rather than dwelling on physical symptoms (Huygen and Smits 1983; Goldberg *et al.* 1989; McDaniel *et al.* 1995). Common experience suggests that there is often more possibility of movement and of helpful understanding for both patients and doctors when people can frame their problems in terms of the difficulties they face in their lives, rather than their subjective experience of malfunction in their bodies. However, in helping patients construct new and more effective stories about what is happening to them, it is usually useful to remain neutral in relation to people's understanding of themselves. The following principles seem to help in this difficult area.

- It is counterproductive to challenge, either overtly or subtly, people's own stories about their symptoms. Until they feel that the doctor has adequately heard their story of having an undiagnosed tumour or intractable ME they are unlikely to be willing to frame their experiences in any other way (Graham 1991).

- If the doctor is hoping for more flexibility from patients in regard to their symptoms, it is also appropriate for the doctor to hold on to the possibility that patients might turn out to be entirely right in their own assessment of their condition. In this respect, it is salutary to bear in mind that we nearly all have patients who died after we or colleagues had given them inappropriate reassurance – and this is exactly what many patients most fear.
- It is often helpful to share the dilemma of making multiple investigations and referrals with the patients themselves. For example, it is possible to say: '*It's relatively easy for me to order another endoscopy or send you to another gastroenterologist if that's what you want, but can we also start to think about what we're going to do if everything turns out to be normal again . . . ?*'

We live in a culture where physical symptoms are often seen as more legitimate than emotional difficulties, and where many people tend to tell stories of their distress in terms of somatic rather than mental manifestations. A very important cultural role for GPs and primary care clinicians may be to listen to these stories without challenging them too starkly, even when there is long-term stuckness. Again, it is possible to check out with the patient whether this understanding of the professional role is helpful for them: '*I'm sorry that none of us seems to have been helpful in making a difference to your symptoms for a very long time. I'm still happy for you to come on a regular basis to let me know what's going on, although we may need to recognise that some things aren't going to change. Would you find that in any way helpful?*' The answer to this question is sometimes yes, and this may produce relief for both the doctor and the patient.

Taking a geneogram or enquiring into the family background can be done in a way that does not imply any blame or responsibility, but may reveal a great deal and move the patient's preoccupation away from pain and suffering.

Crisis intervention

People in primary care quite often see individuals or families in crisis. Understandably, the response is often to make a referral to a counsellor, psychologist or psychiatrist (McNamee 1992). However, by the time these appointments arrive, the crisis has 'gone off the boil'. The emotional impetus for change has been lost, and the home situation may have solidified around an intractable symptom or a sense of fatalism. By the same token, there are opportunities for crisis intervention in primary care that barely exist in any other setting. This chapter ends with an account of one such intervention.

Case study: The W family

A GP told this story: 'I have known the W family for ten years. The members of the family I mainly see are the mother and the daughter Mary, who is now 17. Her parents divorced when she was three. Mrs W subsequently remarried and had two further children, a boy now aged eight and a girl of five.

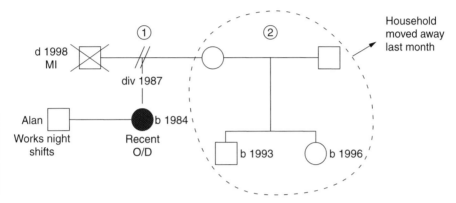

Figure 2   The W family.

'Two months ago, just a week before Christmas, the two women, mother and daughter, came to see me. Mary had evidently taken an overdose the previous week. She had spent three days in a local hospital being washed out and monitored. Mrs W told me that Mary had been seen by the psychiatric SHO and had told him the overdose was because of a row with her boyfriend over the amount of time they spent together. Mary had promised she would not do it again, and the SHO had reassured her mother that it wasn't a very serious attempt.

'When they came to see me, Mary began the consultation crying. She said she had recently moved away from the family home to live with her boyfriend. The boyfriend – Alan – works night shifts as a baker. She finds the long evenings alone frightening, and quite different from what she expected. Her loneliness was worse because recently her mother and stepfather sold the old family home and moved with their two young children some distance away.

'Mary then really started to reproach her mother, in front of me. She accused her mother of spending less time with her in recent months. Then she began to complain how little she had been allowed to see her real father during her upbringing. It emerged that she had only met him five times after her parents' separation when she was 18 months old. He died from a heart attack when she was 14. She talked of how she had been forced to accept her stepfather, and his surname, and of how she had always felt jealous of her half-brother and sister, and less valued than them.

'Her mother seemed to want to explain to me the facts of the situation as she saw it. I asked her to talk about what it had been like as a single mother. She told me she had been deserted by Mary's father. Before that her husband used to spend most of his time and nearly all their money in betting shops. She explained that after the separation he never used his right to have contact with his daughter. She also said that, to her mind, her present husband could not have been more thoughtful about Mary's upbringing.

'I tried to move the conversation on. I asked them to compare their different versions. I used questions like ''Do you see things the same way as Mary on this issue?'' and ''Would you like to comment on what your mother has just said?'' For a long stretch of time, I just sat as a sort of a referee while they explained, argued, protested and just listened to each other.

'After about 25 minutes I gave them a description of the problem as I saw it. I talked about Mary's loneliness. I noted her disappointment at her new life, and the various changes in her circumstances. I offered a suggestion that she was having a delayed grieving. I wondered if selling the family home might seem like the final burial of all her hopes about being part of an ideal family. I also told Mrs W that I appreciated how hard her role was. She wanted to support Mary through the bereavement. But she wanted her own past hardship and effort to be acknowledged.

'I saw them again a week later. Mary came into the room relaxed and smiling. They explained what had passed between them. Mrs W had been able to talk about how her first husband abandoned them. Mary had managed to engage emotionally with this. She had also realised how angry and betrayed she felt herself.

'I also did some ''trouble-shooting''. I asked them what they expected would be the next turning points, or changes, in Mary's life. She talked about her boyfriend and the possibility of marriage, but she wasn't sure about that. She said that if he had more confidence he would consider retraining so he could take a job which gave him more time with her. I trod really delicately here, because he wasn't in the room, but I did say I would be very happy to see him and Mary together if they wished. I haven't seen them for three months since then. I do not know if I will.'

Suggested exercises

- Think of a recent consultation with someone who has a psychiatric diagnosis like depression. What does the diagnosis offer them, and what does it withhold from them?

- Think of a patient who consults frequently or whose narrative often seems repetitive and 'stuck'. Make a list of questions you have never asked that person, but which might take the conversation in a new direction next time you meet.
- What resources are available to you in a mental health crisis? Are there ways in which you might consider extending your involvement in these kinds of crises? What would make it possible to do so safely?

An extract from the sources

The practice of 'story-connecting' questions and challenges every level of story that the persons involved have been assuming and equated with the course of their lives. To question and challenge a story, even as one listens respectfully to it, is to introduce unrealised or forgotten connections between that story and the stories and events which, as seemingly unconnected, have left the person experiencing guilt or powerlessness as she attempts to make her story proceed according to her intentions.

An approach of questioning and challenging within an attitude of validating the person's point of view comprises the hermeneutic stance of the therapist. Intrinsic to the validating role of the therapist with respect to the person finding her voice, is that of offering within a series of challenging, yet respectful conversations, words that give voice to hitherto inchoate experiences. Such words are never imposed from some 'knowing' point of view, but put forth as if only to demonstrate that such experiences can be described and shared through the 'magic' of language. In the give and take of such conversation, the person may gain the confidence to find her own words to her experiences. If such therapy is to be understood as a literary genre, it could perhaps be called conversational autobiography.

Alan Parry (1991)

References

Anderson H and Goolishian H (1992) The client is the expert: a not-knowing approach to therapy. In: S McNamee and K Gergen (eds) *Therapy as Social Construction*. Sage, London.

Armstrong D (1996) Construct validity and GPs' perceptions of psychological problems. *Prim Care Psychiatry*. **2**: 119–22.

Bracken P and Thomas P (2001) Post psychiatry: a new direction for mental health. *BMJ*. **322**: 724–7.

Cooksey EC and Brown P (1998) Spinning on its axes: DSM and the social construction of psychiatric diagnoses. *Int J Health Serv.* **28**: 525–54.

Dowrick C (1992) Why do the O'Sheas consult so often? An exploration of complex family illness behaviour. *Soc Sci Med.* **34**: 491–7.

Goldberg D, Gask L and O'Dowd T (1989) The treatment of somatisation: teaching techniques of reattribution. *J Psychosom Res.* **33**: 689–95.

Graham H (1991) Family interventions in general practice. *J Fam Ther.* **13**: 225–30.

Gremillion H (1992) Psychiatry as social ordering: anorexia nervosa, a paradigm. *Soc Sci Med.* **35**: 57–71.

Hauerwas S (1993) *Naming the Silences: God, medicine and the problem of suffering.* T and T Clarke, Edinburgh.

Heath I (1999) Commentary: There must be limits to the medicalisation of human distress. *BMJ.* **318**: 440.

Huygen FJA and Smits AJA (1983) Family therapy, family somatics and family medicine. *Fam Sys Med.* **1**: 23–32.

Launer J (1998) Narrative in mental health in primary care. In: T Greenhalgh and B Hurwitz (eds) *Narrative Based Medicine: dialogue and discourse in clinical practice.* BMJ Books, London.

Mathers N, Jones N and Hannay D (1995) Heartsink patients: a study of their general practitioners. *Br J Gen Pract.* **45**: 293–6.

McDaniel S, Hepworth J and Doherty W (1995) Medical family therapy with somaticizing patients: the co-creation of therapeutic stories. *Fam Proc.* **34**: 349–61.

McNamee S (1992) Reconstructing identity; the communal construction of crisis. In: S McNamee and K Gergen (eds) *Therapy as Social Construction.* Sage, London.

Middleton H and Shaw I (2000) Distinguishing mental illness in primary care (editorial) *BMJ.* **320**: 1420–1.

Parry A (1991) A universe of stories. *Fam Proc.* **30**: 37–54.

Salinsky J and Sackin P (2001) *How Are You Feeling, Doctor? Identifying and avoiding defensive patterns in the consultation.* Radcliffe Medical Press, Oxford.

Shepherd M, Wilkinson G and Williams P (1986) *Mental illness in primary care settings.* Tavistock, London.

Summerfield D (2001) The invention of post-traumatic stress disorder and the social usefulness of a psychiatric category. *BMJ.* **322**: 95–8.

Wright AL and Morgan WJ (1990) On the creation of 'problem' patients. *Soc Sci Med.* **30**: 951–9.

CHAPTER 7

What hinders narratives

'Descriptions change what is being described.'
Arist von Schlippe (2001)

This chapter examines some common hindrances that impede narratives of all kinds and looks at how to overcome these.

Key ideas in this chapter

- Many practitioners report that they have habits that inhibit patients from developing helpful narratives, and also some ways of encouraging effective new stories.
- Many clinicians appear to have a preference for targeting strong emotions or seeking psychological explanations, but these can impair narratives.
- It is possible to notice common obstacles to narrative development and to finds ways of avoiding these.

Points to consider

- Do any of the hindrances ring bells for you?
- Are there other hindrances that you notice for yourself or others when eliciting narratives?
- How are the suggestions for avoiding these similar to what you do already? Are there other suggestions that you think might help other colleagues to avoid common narrative hindrances?

Hindrances and their origins

Many doctors and nurses report that they have some ingrained consulting habits. These make it hard for them to track the narrative thread of a conversation closely or to draw it out further. This is sometimes true even when they are highly trained and experienced, or when their explicit intention is to behave in a way that is non-paternalistic and empowering towards patients. Even people with additional training in 'patient-centred' approaches, consultation skills or counselling still report that they notice habits in themselves that stand in the way of the patient's narrative.

There may be all kinds of reasons for this. The habits may represent conventional interviewing styles that are widely used in the world of medicine, but seem to impair either listening attentively or giving appropriate responses. Similarly, training in many consultation approaches may not pay precise attention to the micro-skills needed for co-creating narratives with patients.

The following examples demonstrate a number of hindrances that people have reported, or that we have observed in videos or role play. What they all share is that the interviewer in each instance is following an assumption at odds with the ideas and language that are actually emerging. The examples are each followed by suggestions of how to avoid or overcome the particular pitfall illustrated. The examples of conversations are fictional ones, invented for training purposes only.

Not following feedback

Interviewer: When did the problem start?
Patient: As soon as I came back from my holiday.
Interviewer: When exactly was that?

This conversation represents a missed opportunity. By sticking rigidly to the bald facts of chronology, the interviewer has missed something that might be highly important. What is the significance of the holiday in the patient's way of thinking? Could something have happened on the holiday that gave rise to 'the problem', or was it the effects of coming back that may have been associated with it? Are there lessons to be learned from what has happened after previous holidays, or previous returns? Of course, there might not be, but the interviewer will never know without asking circular questions such as these.

Not tracking language

Interviewer: Did the pills make a difference?
Patient: Yes, to quite an extent.
Interviewer: Good, so shall I give you some more?

In some ways, this is a subtler version of not following feedback. What the interviewer is missing here is the precise nuances of language. He has chosen to accept the part of the patient's utterance that is positive, but ignored a more ambiguous phrase ('to quite an extent'). If unpacked, this phrase might turn out to disguise considerable reservations about the treatment. What, in the patient's perception, is the gap between the actual effect of the pills and the desired one? How much might an enquiry into this gap reveal that the patient's initial positive tone arises from diffidence, respect or fear, rather than frankness? Interestingly, one notices these nuances far more as an observer than a participant in an interview. It is also interesting that being observed by one's peers, or frequent experience of being an observer, appears to hone people's ability to be attentive to language and to reflect on an appropriate response.

Being wedded to your hypothesis

Interviewer: Does any particular thought come into your mind before you get a panic attack?
Patient: I don't think so. No.
Interviewer: Try to remember. It's quite common for these things to be triggered off by certain thoughts.

Practitioners often have quite strong beliefs about the nature and origins of particular problems. They are often so concerned to establish that their hypotheses are the correct ones, that they may find it quite difficult to notice when a patient is puzzled or even affronted. Naturally, there are some instances where it is appropriate to probe beyond an initial rejection of a hypothesis. Indeed, a patient might come to agree that a hypothesis that was once strongly rejected was in fact true. On the other hand, pushing a hypothesis too hard can alienate the patient. It may be better to let a previous hypothesis go if it appears to have no use for the patient sitting in front of you at that moment.

Psychologising

Interviewer: Do you think your bowel pattern is affected at all by stress?
Patient: I really don't think so. It seems to be much more related to what I eat.
Interviewer: Yes, but I am aware that you do find your job very stressful at the moment.

Probably the commonest form of being wedded to a hypothesis is psychologising. Contrary to what one might expect, doctors seem to be far more prone to pinning psychological explanations on physical conditions than vice versa. This is probably a manifestation of the widespread modernist belief that everything must have 'an underlying cause' and that psychological underlying causes are somehow more important and profound than anything else (Kirmayer 1994). This may in some cases be true, but what is often problematical is the clinician's implicit claim to know that this is the case even in the face of the patient's clear assertion that it is not. Such a claim privileges the clinician's assumptions over the patient's language and can potentially lead to an abuse of power.

Dwelling on emotions, especially negative ones

Interviewer: How do you feel about having had a stroke?
Patient: Bloody awful at the time, but I'm feeling a lot better now that my strength has come back.
Interviewer: But you must have felt very frightened and angry at first.

Both medical and popular culture during the past few decades have encouraged the expression of strong negative emotion, often on the assumption that it will lead in almost any circumstances to catharsis and relief. Our own observation is that this is very rarely the case, unless it is done with great skill and in protected therapeutic settings. Far more often, we see a rather unfocused attempt to summon or recreate painful feelings in a consulting context, where issues of timing, resources or the other tasks that need to be addressed mean that this is inappropriate. The problem with such attempts is that they allow the patient no choice as to whether they want to explore feelings of this kind. While there may be some occasions when they do wish to express or discharge strong emotion, there is always the danger that they may feel obliged to respond in this way against their will. One way of avoiding this is to pose the choice neutrally, with a question such as: '*Do you want to talk a bit more about how it felt at the time, or would you prefer to say where you are now?*'

Many practitioners seem to fall back on the question '*How did you feel about that?*' when they cannot think of anything else to say (or because they have a belief that delving 'deeper' will eventually reveal 'the truth'). In practice, the question often seems to halt the progress of the narrative by amplifying the negative feelings connected with the problem rather than seeking a way forward. A preferable question may be: '*How would you say you feel about that?*' People may experience this as less intrusive. It may also encourage some reflective distance between themselves and their feelings. This in turn may make it possible for the description, and hence the feelings themselves, to change.

Unsolicited interpretations

Patient: I really lost my rag with my boss last week and I am in pretty deep water as a result.

Interviewer: Did he remind you of someone from your past like your father?

Snippets of psychological theories have made their way into general practice and they are sometimes used in fairly 'wild' ways. The commonest error, as here, is to assume that anything that elicits strong feeling must refer back to someone else from the past, probably a parent. (Incidentally, professionals also tend to do this to each other when consulting on cases, for example suggesting that a particular patient has been upsetting because of triggering unpleasant personal memories. This is discussed further in Chapter 8.) Clearly, there are instances where this is precisely the case, but it is usually more appropriate to ask patients to propose their own hypotheses concerning the causes of problems – rather than jumping on a potentially raw nerve with both feet.

Giving thinly disguised advice

Interviewer: Had you thought of telling your mother you can't visit so often?

Patient: No, not really, I don't think she should cope.

Interviewer: But how would you know unless you tried saying it?

The advice about not giving advice is now thoroughly embedded in the training of many people in primary care. Certainly, most practitioners nowadays are sophisticated enough to know that they must not tell people what to do. On the other hand, the temptation to give advice is irresistible, and it is fairly easy to find ways of giving advice that are not very subtly disguised in the form of questions. Once again, there may often be a place for exploring how different options could be tried out, but this may best be done in neutral forms of words which implicitly give the patient as much permission to reject as to accept the advice. For example, in the case above, it would be possible to enquire:

- *'What effect do you think it would have if you told your mother you were going in less?'* or
- *'How would she show that she wasn't really coping with the prospect of reduced visits?'*

The issue of how to incorporate medical advice has been discussed in Chapter 4.

Compulsive explaining

Patient: I've never really understood what angina is.
Interviewer: Well, let me draw you a picture of the coronary arteries first
                    of all . . .

Many practitioners are thoroughly committed to an educational approach in
their everyday work. They may see explanations as intrinsically empowering
and therefore an essential part of every encounter with a patient. However,
explanations can be problematical, as this example shows. They may pre-empt
any attempt to elicit the patient's own understanding first. For example, does
the patient here really have a mental image or explanatory idea about angina
that might be worth exploring first? Has anyone attempted an explanation to
this patient previously and, if so, what led to the current state of bewilderment?
Often, interviewers give accounts of diseases and treatments in a way that is
well meaning, but simply does not relate to the recipients' levels of understanding, their capacity to take in information or their anxiety. Explanations that are
unrelated to feedback can be oppressive.

The wish to change people

Patient: I really need something for the pain in my knees.
Interviewer: Well I have mentioned before about the importance of losing
                    weight.

There is universal acceptance that doctors, nurses and other health professionals have an important role in disease prevention and health risks. At the
same time, people are often ill-equipped to manage conversations with patients
who cannot change or do not want to. The example here shows an interviewer
who is unable to respond to the fact that previous advice about change has not
been effective. As a result, he does not acknowledge the statement that something is 'needed' (presumably here and now), except with an implied reproach.
What is missing is a frank negotiation about what is possible and why, and
what is impossible and why.

Imposing the professional agenda

Patient: I've really just come for my pills. I'm doing fine generally.
Interviewer: Yes. I see that we haven't done your blood pressure for a
                    while, and we really need to get your cholesterol checked . . .

There is nothing wrong with following good evidence-based medical practice. The failure here, however, is one of contextualisation. The interviewer misses a cue for congratulating the patient on being fine and ignores the possible implication that the patient might prefer having a repeat prescription only. Even if the clinician needs to monitor the blood pressure, cholesterol and so forth, there is no attempt to set it in a meaningful context.

There are no doubt many occasions when doctors need to be able to convey the message: 'I can see that you want to leave, but I am worried about your health'. The problem is that many practitioners report that they find it difficult to be straightforward about this. Instead, they just override the patient's wishes.

On other occasions, a kind of manipulation goes on. The doctor tricks the patient into having something done: for example, checking blood pressure in order to fulfil a quota for audit or income purposes while making it seem as if there is a clinical need. Here too, people find it hard to strategise openly by saying: 'I'm sorry to suggest this at an inappropriate moment, but part of my job is to make sure these things get done . . .'.

Suggested exercises

- After a consultation, try to recall the most productive question or statement that you made and the least productive one.
- When you are not too busy, observe yourself in a series of consultations. Which of your conversational habits slow down people's stories and which of them help the stories flow more freely?

An extract from the sources

Taking narrative seriously will require increased attention to spoken as well as unspoken communication between physician and patient. The metaphors employed by each will require much more careful scrutiny. The rituals of the encounter will require explicit study. To the committed advocate of the purely biomedical model, it will seem as if scientific physicians are being asked to embrace precisely those aspects of 'good bedside manner' that have usually been associated with quacks – people who were forced to employ as pleasing a manner as possible because they lacked any scientific tools for healing – rather than with legitimate physicians.

Is this conscious employment of ritual, metaphor, and story telling, not insincere, fraudulent, or manipulative? The answer will lie both in the physician's assessment of the scientific evidence that supports the efficacy of symbolic modes of healing and in the physician's attitude towards this behaviour. It might well be that the narrative approach will degenerate into a shallow pose if it is employed merely as a tool in the interview, in the way that one might use, for example, an alcoholism screening questionnaire. While the approach might represent a sincere attempt on the physician's part to develop over time into a certain sort of person – a healing sort of person – for whom the primary focus of attention is outward, toward the experience and suffering of the patient, and not inward, towards the physician's own preconceived agenda. As Warren Thomas Reich has argued, 'the litmus test of the sincerity of this approach will be the extent to which the physician becomes vulnerable to a compassionate and empathic experience of the patient's suffering'.

Howard Brody (1994)

References

Brody H (1994) 'My story is broken: can you help me fix it?' Medical ethics and the joint construction of narrative. *Lit Med.* 13: 79–92.

Kirmayer L (1994) Improvisation and authority in illness meaning. *Cult Med Psychiatry.* 18: 183–214.

von Schlippe A (2001) Talking about asthma: the semantic environments of physical disease. *Fam Sys Health.* 19: 251–62.

CHAPTER 8

Clinical supervision

'Clinical supervision or even a bartender's advice can serve the same purpose: to help when the therapist's and family's prejudice enter into a deadly
escalation in search of the "correct" prejudice.'
Gianfranco Cecchin, Gerry Lane and Wendel Ray (1994)

All the chapters so far have focused on one kind of encounter – the consultation
between a practitioner and a patient or patients. This chapter and the next one
look at how to apply a narrative-based approach to work with other professionals. This chapter looks at clinical supervision. The next one looks at work
consultancy.

Key ideas in this chapter

- When practitioners help each other to think about cases, it can improve
  clinical care. It can also help practitioners to develop their overall skills
  in questioning and reflection, and boosts their morale.
- In a complex and demanding field like primary care, many people feel
  they might benefit from clinical supervision, but few receive it.
- Practitioners can learn how to carry out supervision with their colleagues, so that they can help with cases either one to one or in groups.
- Narrative concepts and techniques may work just as well in supervision as in clinical work.

Points to consider

- What are your own sources for help with difficult cases? What are the
  strengths of these sources and what are their limitations?
- How far are the approaches described here realistic in your work setting, or how might they be adapted to make them practical?
- Is there someone you could call on to become you regular supervisor, or
  perhaps for taking turns in developing co-supervision?

Clinical supervision and the culture of primary care

In professions like social work, counselling and family therapy, it is usually considered unethical and possibly even dangerous to work without supervision on one's clinical cases, either in one-to-one discussions with a colleague or in regular, structured clinical team meetings (Carrol 1996; Scaife 2001). Yet in the primary care professions there is no official requirement for clinical supervision, nor any established provision for this. In fact, many practitioners in primary care, on hearing the term 'supervision', understand it to mean something of a managerial or even disciplinary nature. They may be surprised to hear of its other meaning: some protected space, time and peer support for non-judgemental reflection on specific clinical cases. The gap in understanding is striking when one considers the complexity and intensity of work in primary care.

Of course, supervision does exist in various forms in some places in primary care, although it may not go under that name. There are practices and teams where there is an established culture of people talking to each other about their day-to-day difficulties in the consulting room and on home visits. There may also be a regular team meeting to discuss problematical cases on a weekly or monthly basis. In some places, a culture of clinical supervision is beginning to appear among nurses (Morton-Cooper and Palmer, 2000). GP registrars do get time to discuss their cases with their trainers and on their weekly vocational training courses. A number of professionals take part in activities that include an aspect of clinical supervision such as self-directed learning, mentoring, co-tutoring, Balint groups and video review (Jelley and van Zwannenberg 2000; Burton 2001).

However, many people in primary care do not appear to have enough opportunities to talk about cases that are causing them problems of various kinds, especially those that are confusing or distressing them. GPs working in the most depressed and besieged practices seem even less likely than their colleagues to have access to any resources for clinical reflection. Widespread indifference to supervision also seems to be underpinned by a lack of financial and educational resources for the activity. This in turn seems to be echoed by a generally 'macho' culture within some areas of primary care, where clinical anecdotes may be exchanged more as tokens of bravado than as requests for support.

To help to address this lack of opportunity, an important part of our teaching involves giving clinicians the opportunity to carry out supervision with each other, using the same narrative-based approach we teach for the consultation. Feedback suggests that people value sharing their stories about cases, in protected time, and with peers who are applying a narrative-based approach.

Such supervision does not have to take place only with fellow learners on courses such as ours. It can be done by all sorts of people and in various primary care settings. We know of colleagues from individual practices, or from neighbouring ones, who have set up meetings with each other for this purpose – either on an ad hoc basis or regularly. In the course of everyday encounters, GP registrars and alert medical students can provide imaginative case supervision for their trainers, just as much as the other way round. A practice nurse may be willing to offer an alternative perspective by supervising a doctor on some cases. Some practice counsellors or visiting psychologists and psychiatrists may be willing to provide clinical supervision as well as the more conventional kinds of outpatient work in the surgery (Andersen 1984, 1987; Deys *et al.* 1989; Dowling 1994; Rutt and Batchelor 1998). Whatever the combination, two heads are better than one, particularly if the person offering supervision is willing to experiment with developing appropriate skills rather than just trying to solve the problem.

A narrative-based approach to supervision: some principles

The rest of this chapter gives an account of a narrative-based approach to supervision. A number of principles help to make such supervision effective, and these are presented here and illustrated with some cases. The cases here have been adapted from ones that course participants have brought, with enough alterations to preserve everyone's anonymity. In all the cases described here, the clinicians involved were offered supervision with another member of the learning group acting as interviewer, usually with other group members acting as observers.

Narrative-based interviewing can help colleagues in the same way that it helps patients

If patients bring stories that are tentative, incomplete or confused, this is also true of practitioners who are carrying cases that are puzzling or upsetting them. The same disjunctions and hesitancy, repetitiveness and vagueness characterise both. Similarly, narrative-based clinical supervision offers practitioners the same facility that narrative-based practice offers patients. This is the opportunity to present a story and have someone interrogate it intelligently and sensitively, so there is the possibility of a new story. There is often a 'parallel process' between helping the practitioner with a new story and helping the patient with one. In other words, the practitioner who returns to the patient with a far more coherent sense of what is going on and what possibilities there might be for moving the story forward, is far more likely to help the patient to create a more satisfactory new narrative at their next encounter. The benefits of this process may also extend more widely – to more imaginative conversations with patients generally.

Narrative-based supervision has a ready-made methodology, just like narrative-based consultation. A colleague using a narrative approach can employ the same ideas of curiosity, co-construction and so forth, and the same techniques of hypothesising and questioning that would normally be brought to bear in clinical work. These same techniques will also serve to bring out a new understanding of the case with a professional.

To begin with, it is usually easier to practise effective narrative-based supervision in one-to-one encounters. Later, a narrative approach can perhaps be used in group meetings or team sessions as well, but this may require some discipline or team training. Groups can easily veer in the direction of a formless discussion, with everyone bursting to offer advice or suggestions, so that the benefits of careful supervision become lost. (In our teaching, we invariably introduce people first to the skills for supervising each other individually on cases. Only later do we encourage discussion of cases in a large group. This and other training issues are discussed in Chapters 10 and 11.)

Colleagues want to be treated as clients, not patients

A case discussion with a colleague is not the same as a consultation with a patient. This point is worth emphasising because doctors and nurses can have ingrained ways of talking with patients that they then carry over into clinical supervision with each other. For example, they may be used to firing factual questions at speed, or giving advice, or presenting themselves as experts. These habits appear inappropriate when transferred to clinical supervision, which needs a more measured and facilitative style of questioning.

There is inevitably a place for advice and expertise in supervision, just as there is in clinical work. Some people will genuinely have more experience of particular kinds of case than their colleagues and it would be purist for them to withhold good ideas. However, there are a number of helpful guidelines that can protect supervisors from appearing too bossy. One is not to offer advice or suggestions too early in the supervision session. It is often helpful to seek permission before offering advice (for example, with a question like: 'How helpful would it be at this moment if I suggested a possible way forward?'). Advice can also be repackaged within a series of graded questions to test the water and see if the colleague might find it helpful ('What do think would happen if you tried . . . ?') The most important safeguard in this respect is to follow feedback from case presenters and to notice when they want to continue explaining the difficulties of the case rather than be told what to do.

It often helps to start a conversation about a case by asking what the presenter would like help with or any particular kind of focus they would like the interviewer to have (for example, 'I have the feeling I'm missing something important, but I'm not sure what.') It also helps to ask at the end what the presenter got out of the session (if anything), what ideas have been most useful, which questions the practitioner would now like to ask the patient at their next meeting and which options seem the ones most likely to be worth pursuing clinically.

A case discussion can require considerable tact, possibly even more so than most clinical consultations. The clinical, legal and moral responsibility for the case lies with the colleague who is the 'client', and it will continue to do so. The complexity of the case and the levels of distress involved may be greater than the presenter has been able to convey. Colleagues can never assume that they would necessarily handle the case better in real life themselves. Any decision made about how to take the case forward must rest entirely in the presenter's hands.

Case study: A case of pelvic pain

A GP brought a case to a course group involving a patient with a long history of pelvic pain for which no cause had ever been found. The GP was very unsure how to go forward with this woman, who consulted often. A colleague agreed to interview the GP about the case and did so mainly by asking questions. What became clear through the questioning was that the GP felt sure the patient was depressed, but over two or three years had often got into very unproductive discussions with her over this, when she vehemently denied any depression or emotional problems of any sort. He had also offered her antidepressants a number of times to see if it would make a difference to her pelvic pain, but she had refused them. He knew that she was married and did not seem to be very happy with her husband, and on one occasion had asked her directly about her sex life but said she was extremely reluctant to talk about this and seemed to think it irrelevant.

The interviewer widened the discussion to find out if there were areas of her life that the GP did not know about, or which he might be curious to enquire into. It also became clear that the overwhelming emphasis on symptoms and diagnosis had prevented the GP from asking about a wide range of other issues, including her work, her wider family and her childhood – perhaps to a surprising extent, given the nature and chronicity of the problem. With the interviewer's help, he chose a number of areas he might explore to find out more about her and move the consultations away from their usual 'tram lines'.

A month later, the GP reported having had a very productive consultation with the woman. He discovered she had been made redundant as a teacher at about the time the pain started and had been very disheartened at not being able to find another job. He also found out that she had been adopted as a child and was currently engaged in a search for her birth mother. He commented: 'I don't know if any of this will turn out to be relevant, but I think it's probably the first consultation I've ever had with her when she didn't say "Well what's causing it then?" '

Discussing the contexts that surround cases can be more helpful than listening to long descriptions of the cases themselves

Professionals who are stuck with cases are often preoccupied with the precise events of the case: who said what to whom and when, what treatment was given and why, and what happened as a result. Yet when a case is causing difficulty, it nearly always seems to be because there are problems of misunderstanding or muddle in one of the surrounding contexts. It often turns out, for example, that problems have arisen in a case not because of any inherent clinical difficulty but because people in the professional network were in some way working against each other.

For this reason, it is often useful at a very early stage to ask a question like: '*What do I need to know about your work setting that may have a bearing on this case?*' or '*Do you think this case is causing difficulties just between you and the patient or could there be more people involved?*' Such questions focus more quickly on the crux, or potential crux, of the story. They may also draw attention to a possible contextual problem that had been paralysing everyone but had gone unnoticed. Clearly, there needs to be a balance between eliciting too much detail in a case and eliciting too little. A clinician who gets no chance to spell out the bare bones of the case is likely to feel deprived. On the other hand, going into great detail can waste valuable time and prevent a different kind of story ever emerging.

> **Case study: Asthma and the hospital consultant**
>
> A GP spoke about a woman he looked after with severe asthma. A year before, the local chest clinic had discharged her with the instruction 'Just go to your GP and ask for another course of oral steroids when you feel you need them'. This advice was backed up with a letter from the chest clinic consultant, effectively saying the same thing. The patient was now asking for steroids with increasing frequency, sometimes on questionable grounds, but the GP felt constrained from ever saying no. The interviewer moved the focus of the conversation from consultations with the patient on to the relationship with the consultant. She helped the GP to reflect on the way he regarded his own authority as less than the consultant's. With the interviewer's help, he was able to rehearse a possible phone call to the consultant in which he could spell out his story of why the original instruction had created a dilemma for him and ask the consultant to collaborate in producing a more flexible clinical strategy.

Personal issues can be very important for clinicians but need to be handled delicately

Most practitioners have probably had the experience of seeing someone in the surgery who reminded them of people in their own personal lives. They may also have got into difficulties with particular kinds of patients – so-called 'trigger patients' – who caused anxiety, anger and emotional over-involvement. In addition, most would probably have to confess that some patients have excited them sexually, while others have repelled them, made them feel very uncomfortable or reduced them to tears. Such experiences cannot be ignored in case discussions, but they also need to be handled with delicacy, especially in a group or team context.

Because people supervising their colleagues on cases have an apparent licence to ask whatever they want, some are tempted to ask questions like: '*Does this patient remind you of your mother?* or '*Do you find her sexually attractive?*' or '*Have you had an illness like this yourself in the past?*' Most clinicians react with great discomfort to such intrusiveness, feeling quite rightly that they have volunteered themselves for some clinical support from a colleague and not for amateur psychotherapy. Most groups observing people behave in this way also feel that it is inappropriate for the context. There are, fortunately, more subtle ways of moving forward.

The most useful is often to ask a general question about the kind of territory involved without stepping into the territory itself. This means, for example, starting with a general question such as: '*When you think about this case, does it take you into an area that is quite difficult to talk about?*' If the answer is yes, the supervisor can then seek permission to take a small step forward, for example by asking: '*Is it possible for you to say what the area is, or is that something you would rather keep to yourself for the time being?*' An enquiry along these lines does sometimes open up the possibility of taking a gradual series of steps that makes it possible for the client to receive help even in a very emotion-laden case. At the same time, it is vital both for the questioner and the presenter to keep the escape routes open. Case presenters need to know in advance that they are in the driving seat with regard to what they do and do not wish to disclose. They also need the assurance of their colleague that there will be total confidentiality regarding any disclosures.

Clinical supervision is not the only option for help, even with a clinical case. It may be quite appropriate to ask a practitioner: '*If it doesn't seem right to talk about this issue here and now, is there anyone else you might be able to talk to about this?*' Sometimes, the answer to this question is that there is a spouse, or a friend, or even a personal counsellor or therapist whom the client can use as a resource in this way. It is impossible to dodge the issue that some people may show signs of being in considerable personal turmoil during a case supervision or they will disclose that they are dealing with cases where they feel emotionally overwhelmed and out of their depth. Educators, as well as anyone else offering case supervision, need to be prepared to have an entirely private discussion of what help may be needed by the person concerned. Such occasions are rare, but supervision does need to be underpinned by a knowledge of other resources, professional or psychological, to deal with a story that contains more distress than can possibly be explored within a case discussion.

Case study: A case of terminal care

A district nurse brought a case to a course group involving a man with advanced myelofibrosis. His son was insisting that no one should tell the patient or his wife the prognosis and that everyone should just say that he was being treated for a big spleen because some people got that in old age. The nurse felt that this was quite wrong and that patients normally guess what is happening anyway. She found it very hard to be tolerant of the son's view and inclined to override his wishes.

In a case supervision interview, it became clear that the nurse's strong beliefs were very much influenced by personal experience, as her own mother had died from liver metastases after having cancer of the colon. She felt the doctors had been very evasive with all her family and she had resolved never to do so with her own patients. At first she found it difficult to talk about this in front of a course group and became tearful. The tutor intervened to check with the nurse if she wanted the interview to continue. She said she did, as it was important to her to separate her own feelings and experiences from the needs of her job, and she thought the interviewer was being very sensitive. With considerable tact, the interviewer then helped her to think of how to explore her patient's experience or wishes. Quite a long way on in the interview, she admitted that the patient himself had never seemed to be very bothered or curious about his condition. She had also never really had a conversation with the son about who else in the family did or didn't know the prognosis and what he feared would happen if his father found out. The family were also from a different culture and she had not explored with them what would normally happen in their country of origin concerning the open discussion of a poor prognosis.

A lengthy conversation about one case may be more effective than rapidly discussing a series of cases

Among counsellors and therapists it is common for supervision on a single case to last for up to an hour. Given the normal working pace of primary care, and the number of problematical cases that may invite discussion, this can seem like a ridiculous luxury. However, there are a number of good reasons for setting aside reasonable periods of time for discussions with colleagues about a difficult case – probably not less than 15 or 20 minutes – whether in one-to-one supervision or in a group.

First, the longer the discussion about a case lasts, the more chance there is that the person presenting it will change their story from a stuck and repetitive one to a different kind of story where new options have opened up. It is common to hear people express pessimism for the first 10 or 15 minutes of presenting a case, but then they gradually unfreeze and start to develop a new story. Similarly, interviewers may feel as hopelessly overwhelmed as the presenters to start with, but then gradually become more imaginative and flexible in their questioning. The experience of this process, on either side, introduces people to the idea that any case offers multiple possibilities for different approaches, however stuck it might initially have seemed.

Another advantage of a long discussion about a case is that it gives the participants extended practice in conducting such 'conversations inviting change', especially if they are new to this kind of questioning. They can then transfer this experience not only to other conversations with colleagues at work, but also to routine consultations with patients.

Perhaps the most important argument in favour of spending time on a case is that it promotes reflectiveness generally in primary care and therefore acts as a counter to the prevalent culture of telling people anecdotes as the only way of communicating one's distress or difficulties with the work. This is not to deride anecdotes in themselves. They can fulfil an important function in helping professionals to offload their anxiety and stress levels, and perhaps even to seek some simple ideas of how to handle cases in different ways. However, they can also promote a 'coffee room culture' which stereotypes patients and reinforces habits of stuckness. The exchange of anecdotes can also degenerate into a tit-for-tat competition in much the same way that anglers talk about 'the one that got away'. By contrast, experience of prolonged case discussion can potentially influence the work setting so that reflective discussion becomes the norm instead. Although there are many settings where prolonged discussion of this kind may be an occasional luxury rather than a routine, each episode of reflection can lead to a boost in the clinician's ability to manage a difficult case, and perhaps the workload generally, for a period of time.

In time, people do acquire the ability to move faster in thinking about cases, either as supervisors or presenters. Familiarity with circular questioning, and repeated help with difficult cases, leads them to think better on their feet when discussing cases in future. These activities build up people's confidence in making effective interventions in group discussions – for example by framing brief but highly pertinent questions. Such experience also appears to lead to a greater general optimism about cases that might otherwise appear intractable.

Case study: Asking for a referral

A nurse practitioner explained that she ran a hypertension clinic for routine, uncomplicated cases. A 50-year-old man had seen her the previous week. He had recently been diagnosed with mild hypertension and was saying he would rather have his blood pressure checked each time by the GP. The practice's policy was not to do this. She had tried to explain this to the patient but this had led to quite a hostile reaction and left her feeling very uncomfortable. She had felt reluctant to refer the patient back to his GP in the practice to discuss this. A colleague on her course interviewed her and tried to establish what her beliefs were about her work and the hypertension clinic. She said she was very enthusiastic about the clinic in particular. She felt confident running it and belonged to a group of nurse practitioners who were very keen to take over this kind of work. She disliked 'losing' patients back to the GPs and was afraid that they would see any such cases as 'failures' on her part. When the interviewer asked her about the patient's beliefs, she explained he was 'quite a middle class sort of guy' and probably believed that GPs were more reliable than nurses. She was determined to persuade him otherwise and mainly wanted the interviewer to help her think how to do so.

The interviewer then explored various other scenarios if persuasion failed, including 'confrontation' and 'surrender'. This helped the nurse to define a middle position between these two. She decided she would be willing to refer the patient back to the GP with good grace, but first wanted to have a wider discussion with the patient about his views. For example, what things might he be willing to see a nurse practitioner about in future? Also, was there something special about blood pressure (or his worries about it) that had made him so insistent on seeing the doctor?

Suggested exercises

- Next time a colleague wants to discuss a difficult case, offer to set aside some time for peer supervision and use it to practise narrative interviewing.
- When you need help on a difficult case yourself, ask a colleague to interview you about the case, explaining that you want to be questioned rather than advised.
- When you are next taking part in a group discussion of a case, try to make all your interventions in the form of imaginative questions about the case rather than offering information or suggestions.

An extract from the sources

People who have a problem, either personal or professional, tend to be repetitive in their attitudes about the problem. They ask themselves the same questions, and give their questions the same answers. The same answers prescribe the same solutions, and the classical expression '*the attempted solutions become the problem*' comes true.

It would be good for such a person to be supplied with some new ideas, to understand and meet the problem somewhat differently. New ideas, however, are most convincing if they come from the person himself. That occurs when the ideas are answers to questions not usually asked. Such questions must be different enough from the repeated ones to be new, but not so different that they sound bizarre or odd, and not to be taken seriously.

A chart of *both/and* may be of some help. Man is both individual and relational. He has his unique history, will and desires, and he has his courage and endurance to master his flesh and blood. His uniqueness, however, is part of his context which determines heavily how much his uniqueness can be expressed . . . His life, including his context, is connected both to his past and his present and his future; as a human being he also is an oscillating being with both tension and relief, happiness and sorrow, anger and friendliness, activity and rest, boredom and excitement, hope and despair, victory and defeat, connections, disconnections and reconnections, and so on. His context has to respect some space for these individual rhythms for growth and evolution to occur. Just as he goes through his breathing rhythm from inspiration to expiration to inspiration, he should fluctuate through all the other rhythms of mood and activities.

A simple consequence of all this for the therapist is to ask people with a problem one or more of the questions they do not usually ask themselves about those parts of their lives they tend to forget when thinking too much about *either/or*.

Tom Andersen (1984)

References

Andersen T (1984) Consultation: would you like co-evolution instead of referral? *Fam Sys Med.* **2**: 370–9.

Andersen T (1987) The GP and consulting psychiatrist as a team with 'stuck' families. *Fam Sys Med.* **5**: 486–91.

Burton J (2001) Appraisal, supervision and mentoring. *Educ Gen Pract.* **12**: 139–43.

Carrol M (1996) *Counselling Supervision: theory, skills and practice.* Cassell, London.

Cecchin G, Lane G and Ray W (1994) *The Cybernetics of Prejudices in the Practice of Psychotherapy.* Karnac, London.

Deys C, Dowling E and Golding V (1989) Clinical psychology: a consultative approach in general practice. *J Roy Coll Gen Pract.* **39**: 342–4.

Dowling E (1994) Closing the gap: consulting in a general practice. In: C Huffington and H Brunning (eds) *Internal Consultancy in the Public Sector: case studies.* Karnac, London.

Jelley D and van Zwannenberg T (2000) Peer appraisal in general practice: a descriptive study in the Northern Deanery. *Educ Gen Pract.* **11**: 281–8.

Morton-Cooper A and Palmer A (2000) *Mentoring, Preceptorship and Clinical Supervision.* Blackwell, Oxford.

Rutt G and Batchelor H (1998) The doctor, the patient and the supervisor. *Educ Gen Pract.* **9**: 509–11.

Scaife J (2001) *Supervision in the Mental Health Professions: a practitioner's guide.* Brunner-Routledge, London.

CHAPTER 9

Work consultancy

'We all participate as members in a large number of different institutions, of which the workplace is usually one of the most structured and demanding.'
James Mosse (1994)

If primary care professionals have a pressing need to talk about their cases, they often have an even greater need to talk about the problems of their teams and workplaces. This chapter is about such problems, and a way of helping with them. To avoid confusion, the word 'supervision' is used in relation to conversations about clinical work and the word 'consultancy' in relation to workplace issues. In practice, as this chapter will show, the two often overlap.

Key ideas in this chapter

- Professionals in primary care often report that they are more preoccupied with problems in their work setting than they are with clinical cases.
- Providing work consultancy may be a prerequisite for enabling some professionals to work effectively as clinicians, supervisors, teachers or managers.
- Practitioners can help each other with workplace difficulties, either by consulting with someone from their own team or with a colleague from elsewhere.

Points to consider

- Do the kinds of problems described in this chapter fit with your own experience of difficulties in the work setting? What other kinds of problems do you encounter?
- What resources are available to you for helping with such difficulties?
- What additional resources might you be able to find or create?

Work consultancy in action

Sometimes it is reasonably easy for people to discuss their work problems. For example, if someone is experiencing conflict with only one colleague, it may be possible to discuss this in confidence with another member of the team. However, sometimes it is hard to provide such support. Certain people on the team may not be in a position to give unbiased consultancy because they have additional roles as managers or employers – or they may have very strong views themselves about the issues causing concern, so that it is impossible for them to stay neutral. Alternatively, there may be conflict involving many team members, so that everyone is implicated. In circumstances like these, outside help is needed.

This can happen in a number of ways. Local colleagues can act as confidants, providing support for friends or ex-students working on different teams. Some health authorities or trusts provide facilities for 'learning sets', in which local clinicians can discuss their day-to-day working difficulties. Training courses of various kinds, such as our own, also provide safe and supportive settings for this kind of work. Some mental health professionals, especially clinical psychologists and family therapists, are willing to offer time and facilities for this kind of work. Whoever does it, a narrative approach offers one particular way of conceptualising and helping with the difficulties that people come across in their work.

Narrative-based work consultancy: some core themes

A narrative approach to work consultancy is similar to the approach to clinical supervision as described in the previous chapter. The same overall concepts apply. The same questioning techniques are effective. Once again, there is a 'parallel process' at work here. Helping people to create good narratives about their work also helps them to create good narratives with patients. In fact, one of the most compelling arguments for providing professional support for primary care clinicians is that people may not be able to help patients to construct coherent narratives if their own stories as practitioners and team members are shot through with confusions, uncertainties or distress. Nor may they otherwise be able to function fully in all their other roles as team members, teachers, supervisors or managers.

The following account of a narrative approach is centred around some particular examples of workplace difficulties. Rather than focusing on technique as the previous chapters have done, this chapter is organised around a number of themes that usually emerge in work consultancy interviews or group discussions. The main purpose of this is to highlight some of the issues that commonly preoccupy primary care professionals. Another purpose is that it may help to highlight the advantages of carrying out work consultancy in the context of a multidisciplinary learning group.

The cases are all drawn from a number of different courses and workshops we have run in Britain and elsewhere, as well as from consultancy with some practices and teams. They have been heavily disguised in the same way as the clinical cases elsewhere.

Narratives about primary care often describe networks that are complex and unclear

When primary care professionals talk about clinical encounters, they often tell of how these take place in a matrix of professional interactions – in the practice or team, in the health system and in the wider welfare state. Nearly every patient they see is also in contact with some other professional. It may be someone close and obvious, like another partner in the same surgery. It may be someone in a parallel system, like a hospital consultant, midwife or physiotherapist. There may also be people who move in other systems more distant from primary care, people with whom health professionals rarely communicate, but who nevertheless are dealing with the same problem in the same person. These may include, for example, school teachers, police, clergy, benefits agencies, social services, housing departments, insurance companies, lawyers, probation officers, alternative and complementary practitioners, refugee organisations, charities and self help groups. The list is endless.

Primary care workers therefore seem to be acutely aware that their job involves not just managing the interaction with the patient or family. It also means managing a huge range of interprofessional interactions and making sure that the combined effect of these is to produce a coherent and self-confirming story for the patient rather than one that is full of overt or implied disagreements. Some of these interactions will need to be managed directly, by personal contact or phone. Some have to be managed indirectly, by taking care regarding what is said to the patient – in the knowledge that this will be reported to the other agencies involved, and perhaps checked out with them as to its correctness or consistency in the wider scheme of things. Often, people in primary care may be trying to 'second guess' another, unknown practitioner in order not to create disharmony.

One story we hear from practitioners of all kinds is of the existence of barriers and failures of communication between different health professionals.

Optometrists and pharmacists tell us of GPs who never respond to their communications and queries. GPs talk of sending referrals into a 'black hole' (or 'like putting a message in a bottle and throwing it into the ocean'). Narratives from primary care acknowledge the inevitability of such alienation and fragmentation, particularly in the inner city, but also speak of regret. On the one hand, practitioners cannot know and speak to everyone. On the other hand, multi-agency involvement and professional isolation can make the patients' difficulties much worse, especially when the people looking after them are pulling in different directions or are implicitly contemptuous of each others' roles.

Historical events also play a large part in narratives about networks. Doctors bring stories about partnerships that have grown in response to immediate clinical pressures year upon year, or as a reaction to the personal and family needs of individual doctors. Similarly, people talk of how their primary care team or network has expanded for specific historical reasons, perhaps because of an alliance that has built up in the past with a particular individual. Usually, not everyone within a network knows why it functions the way it does or has been a willing participant in the process.

Although much public discourse in primary care emphasises the importance and positive value of teams, the private narratives of individual professionals often belie this, with accounts of divisions and tension. We prefer the word 'network' to 'team', because most work settings in primary care actually involve a number of connected groupings, some quite clear but others less so (Pearson and Jones 1994). GPs, for example, may see themselves simultaneously as members of a partnership, a medical team, a clinical team that includes nurses, a practice team including clerical and administrative staff, and an ill-defined multidisciplinary group with attached health professionals like health visitors and mental health nurses. Some of these groupings may function coherently and harmoniously, but very often this appears not to be the case, as the following case illustrates.

Case study: Getting 'attached' to two practices

A district nurse explained to a course group that she used to cover a geographical patch where her patients were registered with a number of different GPs, some she regarded as good and some as bad. Following a recent policy decision by her managers, she and her colleagues had each been assigned to one or two particular GP practices. She now found herself attached to two sole practitioners, one of whom seemed to have no knowledge of her connection to him. She told of how she had approached him a couple of weeks previously to ask if she could discuss a few cases that concerned her, but he said he did not have the time. She also described how he had passed her in the street a few days after this without even recognising her. The course group gave her an opportunity to speak about her frustration and sense of insult, and also to explore the different options open to her. She decided to take the story back to the managers who had made the original decision, asking them to follow it through with sufficient GP liaison to make it work. She recognised that this might still not have any impact on the GP in question, leaving her with a difficult choice for the future: to ask for a transfer, to grin and bear it, or to resign.

Professionals' stories often refer to a lack of clarity concerning roles and responsibilities

Primary care professionals often speak of their ignorance of other colleagues' roles or responsibilities. Any knowledge they have may be based only on casual contact and vague impressions, or it may be tinged with prejudice. One way that this shows itself is in narratives of unrealistic expectations. Many stories involve interdisciplinary misunderstandings or disappointments. People tell of being asked to do things that they feel are inappropriate to their professions or their particular jobs. Colleagues may have views of their roles that are either idealised or denigratory.

One area where this seems prevalent is in relation to 'minority' professions such as pharmacists, optometrists and dentists. Most people in 'mainstream' primary care appear to regard these as peripheral. Yet they see themselves as having a central role. They speak of how their location on the high street makes them more accessible, and therefore potentially more influential, than professions with higher profiles, and of how they are often consulted over problems of great complexity and seriousness.

One of the commonest narrative themes among primary care clinicians concerns mutual incomprehension and conflict with social services departments. As a result, conversations about work difficulties often have to explore mutual stereotypes. Interviewers may need to seek different descriptions and hence different perceptions.

Case study: An encounter with social services

A GP told her multidisciplinary course group that she was concerned about two under-fives whose mother sometimes appeared to be drunk. She had made a referral to social services but then heard nothing for several weeks. Eventually she had had a phone call from social services inquiring about the 'level of surveillance' she was currently maintaining with the family. She felt this was an inappropriate inquiry, but also felt guilty that she had scarcely seen the family since she originally made the referral. The course group helped the GP to think about her role and responsibility in relation to this family. She decided to seek her practice's support before contacting the social worker once again, in order to explain that GPs do not have any formal right to carry out 'surveillance' of families, and to request that the social services department should conduct a proper investigation.

Networks are opportunities for generating multiple stories. This can be both problematic and creative

As the introduction to this book mentioned, one of the advantages of primary care is that it provides a space for people to explore and create multiple narratives. Patients can try out different ways of reframing their experiences with different members of the team. However, there are also problems with multiple stories. Certain versions of the story brought by the patient may become privileged, while others are devalued, and this can be a source of frustration. This happens especially when the story the doctor hears or remembers becomes the canonical one, while others are disqualified because they are recollected by less-exalted team members. Another problem is that stories from the same patient can be so contradictory or discordant that clinicians begin to feel wary that they are being played off against each other, or set at odds.

Crucial to the management of multiple stories is the practice or team approach to confidentiality. Issues of confidentiality within team contexts have been thoroughly explored (Launer 1994; Waskett 1999), but it seems that mature professionals all recognise that there is a sensible balance to be struck between loose talk and rigid secrecy. Most patients who come to primary care know and expect that there will be some exchange between team members of the information they bring. They may even feel deprived if they feel that no one regards it as being of sufficient importance to pass on to others. Conversely, patients clearly also have a right to privacy, professional intimacy and respect for their autonomy. In this respect, the task of consultancy with a colleague is often to help that person find a way of achieving a balance. It may also be to encourage them to look at wider issues in their work setting, such as whether there are agreed confidentiality codes.

Case study: A dilemma over confidentiality

A pharmacist described to a group of her peers how she had regular contact with a schizophrenic patient who brought in his prescriptions from a nearby GP. Sometimes she knew that the patient was not cashing in his prescriptions, or that he was coming in at long intervals that suggested he was not always taking his medication. Occasionally the patient confessed he had told the GP an untrue story – for example, that he was attending the day hospital or seeing his psychiatric nurse when this was not the case. Recently, she had become aware that the GP had stopped prescribing procyclidine in the past few months. She was unsure if this was an error or intentional, but the patient did seem to be more jittery. Her professional relationship with the GP was good, but she was aware that she had a duty of confidentiality to her customers and did not want to get into a collusive alliance with the GP simply because the patient had a mental health problem. A group discussion helped the pharmacist to clarify in her own mind what would be a legitimate reason for informing the GP. This included her concern about procyclidine, and also any clear evidence that the patient was putting himself or others at risk. However, she felt it would not be legitimate to say that the patient was telling different stories to herself and the GP – something which she recognised anyone had the right to do if they wished.

Differences in power and professional values are crucial in people's stories of their work

People working in primary care often describe how power is concentrated in one particular part of the network – usually the GP partnership, or particular members of it. They also talk of the ways in which this is concealed in the conversations that take place. Partnerships may operate by conflict avoidance and uneasy consensus, or by the habitual domination of one or two individuals in determining decisions. Some never have an open discussion of how older and younger partners rank in relation to each other. Partners may at the same time express a belief that 'everyone is equal' but also say that 'in the end it's the senior partner who really decides'. People from large partnerships speak of how these are 'top heavy', leading to stories of partners who issue contradictory instructions to staff or act unilaterally over issues like workload, holidays or rota duties.

There are many stories of uncertainty over the way GPs and others are expected to relate to each other. Registrars and assistants say they are unclear about their expected roles or their levels of authority. Practices often have no agreed understanding of the difference between directly employed professionals within a GP practice and 'attached' ones, even though the latter are account-able to a different health service hierarchy and are not governed by the doctors' decisions. Receptionists and secretaries offer a particular kind of availability to patients and may have a wealth of important knowledge about them. However, others on the team, especially doctors, may not notice or value this.

A feature of almost everyone's story about their network is a lack of opportu-nity for reflection or seeking clarity about working structures, relationships and values. In spite of the complexity of many primary care work settings, people say it is very much the exception rather than the rule for teams, or discrete parts of teams, to set time aside to reflect on their purposes or how they relate to other groupings. There are often stories about clashes in values between dif-ferent parts of the network, especially the GP partnership and its attached staff. Commonly, GP partnerships are said to be focused on the need to make a profit, while the district nurses and health visitors want to meet specific performance targets based on public health objectives. When providing work support to col-leagues, it is often necessary to explore the history, values and ethos of different disciplines in order to bring out a narrative about collaboration rather than competition.

Case study: Struggling to motivate the GPs

A health visitor took the opportunity of an interview at a training work-shop to express frustration at not being able to motivate the doctors in her practice to screen mothers of new babies in a systematic way for postnatal depression. She contrasted this lack of interest with the doctors' apparent efficiency in immunising the babies themselves. It then became clear that she had a general sense of dissatisfaction at the way that money appeared to dominate the decision making in the practice where she was attached. However, she had only a very vague idea of the system by which GPs are remunerated. Her interviewer, himself a GP, asked her permission to explain something about this, and told her how GP practices that fall short on their immunisation programmes can be financially penalised. In the conversation between them that followed, it became clear that the

GP himself was not aware of the crucial importance that health visitors and their managers place on postnatal depression and its effects on infant mental health. He also had little knowledge of how health visitors are influenced by public health policy and central government directives. The workshop session turned into one of comparing the two different perspectives, and ended in mutual learning in which each professional had a chance to understand more of the other's guiding influences and constraints.

Local and national political issues, especially rapid structural change in the health service, have a great effect on professionals and their stories

Perhaps every generation feels that it is living through times of exceptional and extraordinary change. Teaching primary care professionals in Britain through the late 20th and early 21st centuries, it has been impossible to get away from the feeling that we and our students have been living at the centre of a succession of political and organisational whirlwinds. The obvious way in which this has affected the narratives of working clinicians has been in their accounts of the ceaseless introduction of new initiatives and new concepts. Language has become almost infinitely elastic, so that everyone's vocabulary is now full of words and abbreviations that did not exist a few years ago. People's working networks have been affected by this too, with the introduction of different tiers of management and the appointment of local officers whose job identities involve liaison, education or reorganisation.

A recurring theme is the difficulty of integrating the timeless work of nursing and medicine, rooted in archetypal patterns of human suffering and healing, with the imperative to take on board the latest political fashion for delivering healthcare. The two discourses – the one apparently eternal and the other more transient – often appear to be at odds with each other. Because of this, most professionals seem to be tempted at times to dismiss the endless cycle of reconfiguration as the product of folly and political self-delusion. This is certainly a common refrain that we hear in narratives from primary care. Yet at the same time, there always seems to be an acknowledgement in people's stories that society has to create some structure, necessarily imperfect and temporary, through which it can apply public funds to the relief of private pain and distress.

Everyone in primary care appears to accept their own responsibility for serving the structure as well as the task, although there is almost universal frustration at the time spent on the former. On the whole, this frustration appears to be greater among people working directly for health service trusts, such as community nursing staff, than it does for the remaining independent contractors like GPs, dentists, pharmacists and optometrists. Within the fully nationalised sector, the culture of audit and accountability, and the sense of persecution this can bring about, seems more prominent in people's minds.

One issue that nearly always figures in people's narratives about their work is their autonomy. Most clinicians in primary care appear to have chosen their work in part because of their perception that it would allow them control over their interactions with their patients or clients. Their stories about their own job satisfaction are altered for the worse when they apprehend that external demands, or external structures, are affecting or even dictating the content of those encounters. We hear a great deal from people in primary care about ticking boxes and filling forms, about satisfying targets at the expense of satisfying patients, about the experience of coming to work in order to 'feed the monster'. Satisfaction for clinicians seems to depend on their ability to contain and manage such pressures, sufficiently to feel that encounters with patients are not excessively tainted by it.

Case study: Trying to promote clinical governance

A south Asian GP working as a sole practitioner attended a 'learning set' of local clinicians involved in primary care trust (PCT) work. He explained how he had recently been elected as a representative to his PCT professional executive. His constituency was largely made up of GPs from similar backgrounds to his own, also working as sole practitioners and practising in traditional ways without much staff support. He realised that his colleagues on the executive, mostly white doctors from large and sophisticated practices, were expecting him to pressurise his peers to accept such things as clinical governance, local formularies, drug budgets and introducing counsellors to practices. At the same time, his peers themselves wanted him to persuade the PCT that most patients do not understand or care about such innovations and simply want the kind of personal service they were currently getting from their GPs. The members of the learning set helped him to think about the way he could use his unusual position, with connections and allegiances to both sides, to help each recognise and harness the other's strengths.

Morale and burnout play a large part in people's stories

It is impossible to say whether the recent period of change in the health service has made the issues of low morale and burnout more conspicuous or more pressing than in previous periods. Perhaps such risks are inherent in the work itself or in the kind of people who elect to do such work. Nevertheless, our subjective impression is that we have been working and teaching during a time when these issues are always in evidence and often to the fore. This has been apparent in the stories that course participants have told about themselves and about others in their workplaces. It has also been apparent in feedback concerning the reasons why people have come on courses in the first place, and in their reports of being able to function subsequently in ways that have made them feel less vulnerable.

All kinds of stories testify to the difficulties people are experiencing in their work in primary care, the effects they perceive this work is having on them and their fears of things becoming unmanageable for them. In a sense, many of the foregoing case stories in this chapter are testimony to the pressures that lead people in primary care to question whether they are in the right jobs, and whether it is fair to themselves and their families to remain in them. Interestingly, in most of the stories we hear where morale is implicitly or explicitly raised, it is intraprofessional issues as much as clinical workload that figures. Conflictual partnerships, arguments over money, disagreements over work distribution, unsympathetic or heavy handed management, arbitrary changes to working procedures: these are the things that commonly lead people to talk about taking sick leave or quitting.

These intraprofessional pressures do not of course exist in isolation. They take place against a background of public demand that many primary care professions say they find almost intolerable. The commonest narrative theme in this respect is of quantity, of exposure to a scale and rate of human distress that people feel would beggar belief outside the world of primary care. For GPs, and also for health visitors and community nurses, short consulting times appear to be manageable if patients bring boundaried problems. They are entirely unmanageable if a session is filled with consultations involving multiple and complex needs. Increasingly, primary care clinicians talk of having many encounters in a single day with such 'high-intensity' patients, each of whose needs may include ones that are medical, surgical, psychological, marital, family, legal, housing and related to immigration. Inner-city clinicians may need to use interpreters for many or most consultations. The proverbial ten-minute consultation slot, barely sensible in any light, can seem like a recurrent outrage with such a caseload. Many narratives contrast the reality of this experience with the perceived unreality of official diktats from local managers or governments concerning guidelines, audit, targets, charters or health improvement plans. Work consultancy may involve looking at alternative narratives where the external pressures can be managed within an overall context of work satisfaction.

Case study: Caught in the middle

A district nurse working as a team manager described to a support group of fellow managers how she felt caught in the middle between her own line manager and the nurses on her team who were working at the 'coalface'. She spoke of being under constant pressure from above to professionalise her workforce by setting quality standards, saying that she was also being encouraged to 'weed out' those who were underperforming – using disciplinary procedures where necessary. At the same time, the message from the nurses in the community was that they were overstretched and demoralised. It was also clear to her that dismissals could only make things worse. Her support group helped her to consider how she might present quality standards to her juniors as a potential source of job satisfaction rather than as hurdles to be jumped over. They also helped her to plan how she could give her line manager a dispassionate story of her team's morale, neither understating it nor appearing to obstruct change. Interestingly, her discussion with the group led her to entertain the possibility that her line manager might himself feel under enormous pressure from the top level of management. He even might appreciate having a well-constructed narrative concerning morale in the workforce in order to justify slowing down the pace of change.

People working in primary care are sustained by personal values and personal relationships, both within their primary care teams and outside

Writing in *Doctors on the Edge*, the narrative researcher Linden West describes how city GPs are sustained not by the official structures of the health service, but by their own individual values and the relationships, both personal and professional, that they have built up around them (West 2001). Working in a postgraduate educational setting, we have found this to be true not only of GPs but also of all their colleagues from other disciplines. Primary care clinicians acknowledge the complexity of motives that took them into their professions, and into primary care in the first place. The motives they describe include not the trite and conventional one of 'wanting to help people', but more often a subtle and changing mixture of family influences, personal experiences, political or religious beliefs, circumstances, ambition and unknown or unknowable factors as well. What keeps them going are friendships in the workplace, the solidarity of a good team, respect for a manager who is herself respectful, and very often the backup of a spouse or domestic partner and a family.

One thing that is striking in the narratives that people in primary care tell about their work is the closeness in their minds between the professional and the personal. In the safe context of a learning group, people may talk both about the work itself and about the personal connections and beliefs that help them to make sense of it. Doctors and nurses who were themselves once refugees or immigrants have spoken of how they apply their own experiences of displacement to working with a later generation of refugees from an entirely different continent. Clinicians from minorities with strong religious beliefs have disclosed how much their community ties and commitment inform their medical work. Gay and lesbian practitioners have explained how marginalisation has sharpened their understanding of many of their patients. People who are parents often refer to the importance of their own experience of raising children and how they apply this experience in their work. Those who have nursed sick or dying parents, or who have themselves been through serious illnesses, have reflected on the way this has changed their own attitudes or practice. While respecting people's sensitivities and allowing them to remain silent, we have also found it important to give people permission to make connections between their professional and personal lives. Doing so is, in a sense, a prerequisite for developing a narrative approach. It opens the possibility of a seamless story that makes sense of what people do in primary care, and why they do it.

Case study: Scroungers or deserving poor?

A discussion in a primary care team concerned particular kinds of patients who were perceived by some to be 'scroungers'. The GPs in the team took exception to this description, saying that it was important to try and understand why certain patients seemed to demand more than their legitimate share of benefits such as disability allowances. They argued that one could never know exactly what patients' subjective suffering might be. These doctors had a political commitment to accepting at face value the account that patients gave of their own needs. They each had a commitment to helping patients suffering from economic deprivation. At that point the two nurses in the team – both with strong Christian beliefs – said that they believed that everyone had responsibilities to society as well as rights. What motivated them in their own work, they said, was a religious commitment to fairness and justice. They expected this from their patients as well as themselves. They said they would not fight shy of making this point to people who seemed to be making exaggerated claims for special consideration. Neither the doctors nor the nurses had been aware previously of the two differing views. They discussed whether both points of view could be held harmoniously within the same team, and came to the conclusion that it was rather healthy that they were.

Suggested exercises

- When a colleague next tells you about a work problem, see if you can offer support through a narrative approach and questioning rather than through sympathy and advice.
- Next time a work difficulty arises, consider how you might approach it from a different perspective. For example, ask a colleague if you can have a confidential discussion to develop your thinking about it. Or use a group setting away from your work place to ask for some independent consideration of the problem.
- If there are mental health professionals in your network who do consultancy work of any kind, consider if it would be appropriate to ask them if they would be willing to act as a resource sometimes to help people in the workplace think about problems wider than clinical ones.

A quote from the sources

There are some areas of primary care where there is little or no literature using a narrative viewpoint. In these cases, we try to write appropriate material to cover the ground, or use work we have published ourselves. This includes the area of work consultancy. The following extract looks at how mental health professionals working alongside primary care might conceptualise their work in a different way.

What might a 'general mental health practitioner' do within a practice or primary care team? They should almost certainly be thinking about crossing some of the conventional boundaries between individual and family case work, training, case consultancy, supervision and perhaps even organisational consultancy. Since the field of primary care is inherently antipathetic to clear categories such as these, attached mental health professionals at least need to be asking questions about how their generic skills can be most useful in the community context, and entering into some kind of dialogue with GPs and teams about this. Inevitably, there will always be practices where no one wants anything other than the 'dry cleaning' model. In such places it may be appropriate to offer just that, although perhaps with some graded and tactful questioning about the stresses that led the organisation to want such a limited engagement with help. At the other end of the spectrum, there may be only a very few practices wanting to use an outside individual for help with everything from casework to assistance with personnel or partnership matters at the other end. Even in these cases there will be important questions to ask about the exact boundaries of the work and whether it is appropriate to combine several functions in the same person.

Yet as mental health services and primary care draw closer, and as managers look more closely at the best use of human resources, there are likely to be challenges to the belief that psychologists, counsellors or mental health nurses are just in the building to see individual patients behind closed doors. Given all the current changes and pressures on the primary care scene, more innovative and evolutionary models of collaborative working may become the norm ... What seems the way of the future, then, is for mental health professionals to be seen and used as resources for thinking and reflection in primary care, and for service development.

John Launer (2002)

References

Launer J (1994) Psychotherapy in the GP surgery: working with and without a secure therapeutic frame. *Br J Psychother*. 11: 121–6.

Launer J (2002) The practice as an organisation. In: J Holmes and A Elder (eds) *Mental Health in Primary Care: a new approach*. Oxford University Press, Oxford.

Mosse J (1994) The institutional roots of consulting to institutions. In: A Obholzer and V Roberts (eds) *The Unconscious at Work: individual and organisational stress in the human services*. Routledge, London.

Pearson P and Jones K (1994) The primary care non-team. *BMJ*. **309**: 1387–8.

Waskett C (1999) Confidentiality in a team setting. In: R Bor and D McCann (eds) *The Practice of Counselling in Primary Care*. Sage, London.

West L (2001) *Doctors on the Edge*. Free Association Books, London.

PART TWO

Teaching

CHAPTER 10

Background

This part of the book is a parallel story to the previous one. It is another way of describing how to take a narrative-based approach, but from a historical and educational perspective rather than in the form of a manual for everyday practice. It can be read as an expansion of the previous section or as an alternative point of entry to the whole of the book. Like the different stories that patients may tell at different times, or to different people, this story describes the same things as before, but at the same time creates a new narrative of its own.

This chapter describes the background to the primary care training at the Tavistock Clinic, and hence to the approach described in this book. The rest of the section describes the training itself and looks at its effects on participants.

The main contexts

To understand how and why the Tavistock training happened, there are several contexts that need to be taken into account. All of these have been alluded to in the Preface and Introduction but they are discussed here in fuller detail. They are:

- the nature of family therapy
- how family therapy thinking has evolved
- links between primary care and family therapy
- what happens in family therapy training
- the role of the Tavistock Clinic in primary care training.

Readers who are familiar with some of these topics may want to skip parts of the chapter.

The nature of family therapy

Most people working in primary care have some impression of what family therapists do, but it may be helpful to start with a clear and simple description of this.

Family therapists see families. They see family members together in twos or threes, or larger numbers. They see families of all kinds. There are no rules about patients having to be married, or a nuclear family, or anything else. There is no prior commitment to persuading families to stay together, or to break up, or to behave in any normative way; that is not the point of seeing them. Sometimes therapists see families together with other people who are involved in their lives, such as their social worker, schoolteacher, health visitor or GP. Sometimes they see parts of families because the other members cannot come or do not want to. They may see individuals, although when they do so the subject of conversation is often their family and their relationships. Quite often there is a series of meetings with different combinations of family members. Family therapy can take place in a single assessment session, or at intervals of a week, a fortnight, a month or more over a long period – perhaps a year or two. Different practitioners and institutions offer different arrangements to families, and obviously will offer a length of treatment in response to the seriousness of the presenting problem.

Family therapists choose to work with families because they believe that the family is usually implicated in anyone's problems. This does not imply that they blame parents, or spouses, or families as a whole, for any individual's set of problems. Instead, they simply believe that every problem has a relational aspect to it. In the development of any one person's problem, other people's behaviour has often played a part. Once that problem has arisen, the response of other family members may intensify it rather than helping. Problems may make more sense as part of an interacting pattern rather than just as a set of symptoms.

Family therapists also see families rather than individuals because they think it may help to solve problems more quickly and effectively. Some families use meetings to discover how to collaborate with each other, whereas they might have pulled in different directions if they had not been seen together. Handled properly, many families find it an important experience to sit down together and have the opportunity to talk to, and with, each other. For some people, it can produce the first active realisation that they are mutually dependent and can be mutually nurturing. Above all, the interview itself may have a therapeutic effect by inviting the family to explore and develop new narratives.

In Britain, the major practical impact of family therapy has been in the field of child and adolescent psychiatry. Most child guidance clinics in this country now include the word 'family' in their names. Many of them have on their teams at least one child psychiatrist, psychologist or social worker who has had additional training in family therapy. Regardless of the particular approach they might take, they all share the premise that children's problems are usually inseparable from wider difficulties within the family and are often best addressed by seeing the family together for joint therapeutic work. To a lesser extent, a couple or family approach is now taken in some parts of the adult mental health sector, in departments of clinical psychology, adult psychiatry and social work (Falloon *et al.* 1993).

How family therapy thinking has evolved

The first person to see the family together for therapy was probably the psychiatrist John Bowlby, working in the 1940s at the Tavistock Clinic (Bowlby 1949). However, as an organised movement, family therapy took off largely in the United States in the 1950s. To a great extent, it originated there as a reaction to psychoanalysis and the psychoanalytic emphasis on the individual and the psyche. A number of psychiatrists moved their attention towards the family and its interactions instead. They drew their ideas from a variety of sources outside the world of mental health, including general systems theory, evolutionary biology, cybernetics and communication theory (Watzlawick *et al.* 1967; von Bertalanffy 1968; Bateson 1972).

At the time of its inception, family therapy was in some ways much closer to medicine than it is now. There was a preoccupation with concepts like structure and homoeostasis, and how these might apply to families (Hoffman 1982). The thinking of family therapists was revolutionary in so far as it saw the world in terms of unceasing interactions rather than in terms of cause and effect. However, it was also quite conservative in the sense that most family therapists, like most psychoanalysts, believed that they had hit upon a form of truth about the way the world operated.

This view led family therapists to formulate certain kinds of descriptions of families. For example, Salvador Minuchin proposed that some families were excessively close or 'enmeshed', while others were 'disorganised' (Minuchin and Fishman 1981). Other therapists employed terms like 'triangulation' for the way a child became caught up in parental arguments. Similar views led therapists to set particular kinds of tasks for families to shake them out of interactions that were seen as dysfunctional. Some, like Haley, set 'strategic' tasks to prescribe new kinds of experiences for families (Haley 1978). Others, like Palazzoli and her colleagues, set 'paradoxical' tasks, often telling people to try and maintain or even intensify their symptoms, to confront families with the illogical ways in which they were behaving (Selvini Palazzoli *et al.* 1978).

Family therapy has never been a monolithic movement. Different practitioners and teams have always worked in different ways, and the number of identifiable schools of thought over the years is probably uncountable (Nichols and Schwartz 2001). A few have sought to draw closer to psychoanalysis again, seeking a synthesis of psychoanalytic and family-oriented approaches (McFadyen 1997). Similarly, a small number have followed Bowlby himself in paying particular attention to the nature of people's attachments (Byng-Hall 1995). This list is far from exhaustive.

In its relatively short history, there have been quite a number of shifts in the overall thinking of most family therapists, whatever their orientation. Two of these shifts have been particularly important. The first was due to the input of new ideas in the 1980s by the 'Milan Team', who identified themselves as 'systemic' family therapists. They and their followers introduced many of the basic concepts and interviewing techniques that we still teach, and that were covered in Chapters 2 and 3. In theoretical terms, their biggest contribution was probably in placing an emphasis on the therapist's neutrality, and in their understanding of the interview as the treatment in itself, quite independent of any formulation or suggestions that might be given at the end (Palazzoli Selvini *et al.* 1980). They also helped to move family therapy forward by inviting therapists to consider themselves very much as part of the 'system' in the room rather than as objective observers.

The next major shift was the so-called 'narrative turn' described in the Introduction (Gergen and Gergen 1986; Brown *et al.* 1996). Under the influence of all kinds of contemporary intellectual and political movements – including feminism, antiracism and, in particular, post-modernism – family therapists became aware of the substantial critiques that were being launched against conventional versions of 'truth'. They became aware of ideas from social sciences, philosophy and the humanities which suggested that an objectively knowable truth was an illusion and that what we believe to be the truth is the product of social agreement only. These ideas coalesced under the name of 'social constructionism' (McNamee and Gergen 1992). Family therapists have defined this in various ways but the following two quotations are representative.

> Social constructionism sees knowledge of the world as made up purely through social communication – reality is what we agree with other people. (Pocock 1995)

> Social constructionism views discourse about the world not as a map of the world but as an artefact of communal interchange. (Gergen 1985)

Views like these have had a revolutionary effect on how family therapists work, in a number of ways. One of these is that it has moved the focus of their work away from the 'system' towards language and narratives. Another is that it has led most therapists to pay far more attention to the voices of those who lack power in the situations in which they find themselves – especially women, people from ethnic minorities, the physically ill and disabled, and people with other disadvantages and deprivations. It has also sensitised therapists to the possible abuse of their own power by practices that might be inappropriately authoritative or paternalistic. It is these aspects of contemporary family therapy thinking that most appealed to us when we set out to think about new ways that family therapy ideas might be transferred to primary care.

A number of other recent trends are also worth mentioning briefly because of their particular relevance to primary care. The Australian family therapist Michael White has promoted a markedly democratic style of work that involves elements such as correspondence with patients by letter. He has also pioneered the use of an approach he calls 'externalisation'. This involves naming troublesome behavioural or emotional problems, such as encopresis or jealousy, as if they are uninvited guests who have intruded on the family and can be managed as such (White and Epston 1990). Other therapists, including Steve de Shazer, have taken a special interest in the place of brief interventions – taking perhaps one or two sessions – as opposed to longer therapy (de Shazer 1985). Finally, there has been a burgeoning interest in outcome studies in family therapy. This has shown encouraging results in a variety of areas, including chronic physical illness and anorexia nervosa (Campbell and Patterson 1995; Dare *et al.* 2001). In depression, family therapy involving patients and their spouses or partners has been shown to be more effective than either medication or cognitive therapy (Leff *et al.* 2000).

Links between primary care and family therapy

There is a long history of GPs who have become interested in family therapy and of family therapists who have become involved in primary care. This section is a brief account of this history.

The doyen among GPs with an interest in family therapy was the Dutch family doctor FJA Huygen. His book *The Medical Life History of Families* (Huygen 1982) is widely considered to be one of the masterpieces of general practice literature. In it, Huygen reported meticulously on the life events and medical history of about 20 families from his practice over three decades. He introduced the idea of the family illness chart, which records how different family members consult over time. He also reported on two studies of 100 younger families and 100 older families, which he subjected to thorough statistical analysis. From his studies, Huygen showed that children were more likely to need the doctor when parents tended to avoid conflict or when they had isolated mothers, parents prone to somatic complaints and a number of other variables. He subsequently became interested in family therapy and was the first GP worldwide to demonstrate a reduction in consultation rates by the whole family after family therapy (Huygen and Smits 1983). Taken altogether, his life work was a milestone in qualitative medical research.

In some parts of the United States, family therapy and family medicine have worked together closely for many years. The drive for this has come from a core of enthusiasts including Don Bloch, Bill Doherty and Susan McDaniel, together with the other founders of the Family Systems Medicine movement. They have consistently argued that primary medical care should be the main setting where work with the family should take place, and that it offers opportunities for effective work with the family that are not offered anywhere else (Bloch 1983, 1987; Doherty and Baird 1983; Dym and Berman 1985, 1986; McDaniel *et al.* 1992; Seaburn *et al.* 1993).

In recent years, the same group of people in the US has founded the Collaborative Healthcare Coalition, promoting increased clinical collaboration between family physicians and therapists as 'integrated primary care' (Blount 1998; Bloch and Doherty 1998, 2001)) The work of this group of people has been largely based on the 'biopsychosocial model' developed by their mentor George Engel (Engel 1980). Engel's model has now had tremendous influence in primary care worldwide (Engel 1996). It has encouraged primary care workers everywhere to consider the emotional and family dimensions of people's problems. It has also led them to take much more seriously the emotional and social effects of illness and disability and to pay these more attention. However, it has also had critics. These have argued that the model encourages doctors in the false belief that they have an 'objective' view of psychological and social realities, and prompts them to abuse their power by intervening in people's family and social lives as well as their illnesses (Armstrong 1987).

One exceptional thinker at the interface between primary care and family therapy has been the Norwegian psychiatrist Tom Andersen, himself a former GP (Andersen 1984, 1987). Working as an airborne consultant to GPs in remote Arctic communities, he has pioneered the use of consultation to GPs who are having difficulties with particular individuals or families. He has also been at the forefront of those who have taken a more narrative approach to people's difficulties and their solutions (Andersen 1992.) In Finland, Pekka Larivaara and his colleagues have shown a particular interest in using family therapy to address the problems of frequent consulters (Larivaara *et al.* 1996). They have also developed primary care training in family systems medicine (Larivaara *et al.* 2000) that has some similarities to the Tavistock Clinic course.

In Britain, a number of individual GPs have been pioneering the cross-fertilisation of ideas between the two fields since as long ago as the 1960s. These have included Ted Hatfield, Peter Tomson and, in particular, Hilary Graham (Hatfield 1995; Tomson and Asen 1987; Tomson 1990; Graham 1991). There have been two distinct strands in their work. One is to explore how GPs can use family approaches such as taking geneograms or asking circular questions in the course of their normal work. The other is to find ways of promoting work with families or couples, either in longer sessions or in dedicated clinics, to address a wide range of physical and emotional difficulties (Graham *et al.* 1992). A number of therapists in Britain have also ventured into primary care. They have explored how to adapt their work to the primary care setting, looking in particular at how to reach the kinds of patients who would not usually consider attending a specialist clinic for therapy or be referred to one (Deys *et al*. 1989; Asen and Tomson 1993; Carpenter 1994; Senior 1994).

In recent years, the Thinking Families Network in Britain has drawn together a wide variety of people who want to explore the ways that primary care can make use of family therapy (Tomson and Czauderna 1994; Launer 1995). Involvement with the Thinking Families Network, and collaboration with many of the people involved with it, has contributed a great deal to the ideas we now teach.

What happens in family therapy training

Our primary care training at the Tavistock Clinic draws to some extent on features from the training of family therapists.

All family therapy training is *multidisciplinary*. Trainees come from a variety of backgrounds, including clinical psychology, social work and psychiatry. In nearly every case, they are acquiring family therapy ideas and skills as an adjunct to their existing professions. Comparatively few trained family therapists go on to practise exclusively in family therapy or to identify themselves exclusively as family therapists. Most choose instead to take up educational, management or consultancy roles within their own professions and workplaces.

The multidisciplinary nature of family therapy training seems to have some distinct effects. It exposes trainees to working with professionals who have complementary skills and forms of knowledge to their own. It therefore enhances understanding and respect between disciplines, and may foster better team working. It also encourages trainees to consider whether clients necessarily find it useful for the different professional disciplines to exist in the rather rigidly defined ways that they do.

It takes four years of part-time training to become a family therapist in Britain, but the majority of people who go on family therapy courses do not join for the complete training. They commonly go for one or two years only, and if they do eventually carry on to complete the qualification, this may only be after an interval of some years. There is widespread recognition in the family therapy world that there is a need to equip very many kinds of professionals with basic skills and ideas in the field, even if they have no intention of ever working as family therapists. The notion has now grown that such people should be encouraged to regard themselves as '*systemic practitioners*', valuing their existing professional talents and wisdom, rather than regarding themselves as incomplete therapists.

Most basic family therapy training consists of *theoretical and case-based learning*, mainly in small group seminars. The level of theoretical learning is often equivalent to that of a Masters' degree, and many courses are now accredited as such. The premium placed on reading and on personal intellectual development reflects a tradition in family therapy of taking theoretical ideas seriously and regarding them as a prerequisite for good practice. Small group seminars also give participants the chance to bring details from their own current caseload to seek supervision from the group. This has the advantage of introducing learners to some of the approaches to supervision and work consultancy, as discussed in Chapters 8 and 9.

Those who proceed to a qualification-level training do all their clinical work in *peer groups*. The same person will carry the clinical responsibility for seeing any one couple or family through their therapy, but the other members of the group and the tutor participate in the therapy in other ways. These include joining in discussions about the case before and after each session, and perhaps in a break in the middle too. They also include observing therapy sessions through a one-way screen or video link, and possibly reviewing the video afterwards. In some cases, members of the group may go into the therapy room as co-therapists, observers or as a reflecting team (*see* Chapter 3).

Why work in this elaborate way? From an educational point of view, it gives trainees opportunities to develop their clinical skills, not only when they are seeing a family themselves but also when they are observing their peers. From a therapeutic point of view, this way of group working generates multiple viewpoints. This can help the couple or family being seen. For example, their therapist may use a question or idea that a colleague has proposed during a break. Alternatively an observer or reflecting team in the room might come up with an idea that the family finds particularly useful.

In our own primary care trainings, we have sought to introduce whatever seemed most practical and helpful from family therapy training and could be sensibly adapted for primary care.

The role of the Tavistock Clinic in primary care training

One remaining context needs to be described briefly in order to provide a background for our work: the Tavistock Clinic.

The Tavistock is a postgraduate training institute for mental health and part of the British National Health Service. It specialises in offering psychological treatments, including individual, group and family therapy. It also provides basic and higher professional training for psychologists, psychiatrists, and family therapists and psychotherapists. It offers clinical and organisational consultancy services to the public sector and other agencies. In addition, it has a tradition of offering part-time 'application trainings' to support front line workers in the health and social services with the whole range of their work.

Many in primary care associate the Tavistock Clinic with the work of Michael Balint (Balint 1957) and therefore mistakenly assume that we are part of the Balint movement. We share Balint's enthusiasm for primary care as a setting where encounters of professional intimacy and effectiveness can take place. However, we differ considerably in our theoretical background, our teaching techniques and in the kind of clinical practice we promote. The people involved in teaching on the primary care course are not psychoanalysts like the Balints. We all belong to a different grouping within the Clinic: the Systemic Psychotherapy Group (Papadopoulos and Byng-Hall 1997). All of us are family therapists, as well as having a core discipline of general practice, child psychiatry, clinical psychology or social work. Our teaching techniques are unlike those of Balint groups, in that we place an emphasis on theoretical learning and specific skills training. The kind of clinical practice we promote is one that is based on social constructionism and an emphasis on language rather than on feelings, the doctor–patient relationship or ideas concerning the unconscious mind. (A fuller comparison of the Balint movement with a narrative-based approach is the subject of Chapter 16.)

The project of developing a new primary care training at the Tavistock evolved in a number of stages. Up to the 1990s, GPs had been represented in running and attending Balint groups at the Tavistock but no GP or primary care practitioner had ever undertaken a training in family therapy at the Clinic. When the author first enrolled on such a training in 1993, it was mainly with a view to learning 'how to do family therapy in a GP setting'. However, it soon became apparent that there was a much more interesting task to address: looking at how skills and ideas from family therapy could be applied to the whole range of primary care work. As a result, the author, together with his tutor Caroline Lindsey, conceived of a research project looking at how social constructionist ideas might be applied to the field of general practice as a whole. This project is described fully in the Appendix.

The research provided a bridge between the theoretical ideas from family therapy and a practical training for primary care. The research findings confirmed our belief that social constructionist ideas might be both powerful and highly useful in a primary care context. They pointed towards a core set of ideas that might form the basis of a practical training course. Most significantly, they suggested that a number of specific practical skills from family therapy could be taught to people in primary care, and that these might enhance practitioners' overall competence and help them to empower patients. As a result, we designed a pilot course and ran this for the first time from January 1995. The course has run regularly ever since. The next chapter provides a broad description of the training we offer, and the subsequent chapters give a more detailed account of its content and its results.

References

Andersen T (1984) Consultation: would you like co-evolution instead of referral? *Fam Sys Med.* **2**: 370–9.

Andersen T (1987) The GP and consulting psychiatrist as a team with 'stuck' families. *Fam Sys Med.* **5**: 486–91.

Andersen T (1992) Reflections on reflecting with families. In: S McNamee and K Gergen (eds) *Therapy as Social Construction.* Sage, London.

Armstrong D (1987) Theoretical tensions in biopsychosocial medicine. *Soc Sci Med.* **11**: 1213–18.

Asen K, Tomson P (1993) *Family Solutions in Family Practice.* Quay, London.

Balint M (1957) *The Doctor, his Patient and the Illness.* Pitman Medical, London.

Bateson G (1972) *Steps to an Ecology of Mind.* Ballantine, New York.

Bloch D (1983) Family systems medicine: the field and the journal. *Family Sys Med.* **1**: 3.

Bloch D (1987) Family/disease/therapeutic system: a co-evolutionary model. *Fam Sys Med.* **3**: 277.

Bloch D and Doherty W (1998) Editorial: The Collaborative Family Healthcare Coalition. *Fam Sys Health.* **16**: 3–6.

Bloch D and Doherty W (2001) Editorial: The continuing evolution of the Collaborative Family Healthcare Association. *Fam Sys Health.* **19**: 1–4.

Blount A (1998) *Integrated Primary Care: the future of medical and mental health collaboration.* Norton, New York.

Bowlby J (1949) The study and reduction of group tension in the family. *Hum Relations.* **2**: 123–8.

Brown B, Nolan P, Crawford P and Lewis A (1996) Interaction, language and the 'narrative turn' in psychotherapy and psychiatry. *Soc Sci Med.* **43**: 1569–78.

Byng-Hall J (1995) *Rewriting Family Scripts. Improvisation and systems change.* Guilford Press, London.

Campbell T and Patterson J (1995) The effectiveness of family interventions and the treatment of physical illness. *J Marital Fam Ther.* **21**: 545–83.

Carpenter J (1994) Older adults in primary health care in the United Kingdom; an exploration of the relevance of family therapy. *Fam Sys Med.* **12**: 133–48.

Dare C, Eisler I, Russell G, Treasure J and Dodge L (2001) Psychological treatment for adults with anorexia nervosa: randomised controlled trial of outpatient therapy. *Br J Psychiatry.* **178**: 216–21.

de Shazer S (1985) *Keys to Solution in Brief Therapy.* Norton, New York.

Deys C, Dowling E and Golding V (1989). Clinical psychology: a consultative approach in general practice. *J Roy Coll Gen Pract.* **39**: 342–4.

Doherty W and Baird M (1983) *Family Therapy and Family Medicine.* Guilford Press, New York.

Dym B and Berman S (1985) Family systems medicine: family therapy's next frontier? *Fam Ther Networker.* **9**: 20–9.

Dym B and Berman S (1986) The primary health care team: family physician and family therapist in joint practice. *Fam Sys Med.* **4**: 9–21.

Engel G (1980) The clinical application of the biopsychosocial model. *Am J Psychiatry.* **137**: 535–44.

Engel G (1996) From biomedical to biopsychosocial: I. Being scientific in the human domain. *Fam Sys Health.* **14**: 425–33.

Falloon IRH, Krekorian H, Shanahan WJ, Laporta M and McLees S (1993) A family-based approach to adult mental disorders. *J Fam Ther.* **15**: 147–62.

Gergen K (1985) The social constructionist movement in modern psychology. *Am Psychol.* **40**: 266–75.

Gergen KJ and Gergen MM (1986) Narrative form and the construction of psychological science. In: TR Sarbin (ed) *Narrative Psychology: the storied nature of human contact.* Praeger, New York.

Graham H (1991) Family interventions in general practice. *J Fam Ther.* **13**: 225–30.

Graham H, Senior R, Lazarus M, Mayer R and Asen K (1992) Family therapy in general practice: views of referrers and clients. *Br J Gen Pract.* **42**: 25–8.

Haley J (1978) *Problem Solving Therapy.* Harper-Row, London.

Hatfield FES (1995) *Understanding the Family and its Illnesses: a system of family psychiatry for general practitioners.* Sue White, Preston.

Hoffman L (1982) *Foundations of Family Therapy.* Basic Books, New York.

Huygen FJA (1982) *Family Medicine: the medical life history of families.* Brunner/Mazel, New York.

Huygen FJA and Smits AJA (1983) Family therapy, family somatics and family medicine. *Fam Sys Med.* **1**: 23–32.

Larivaara P, Väisänen E and Wynne LC (1996) Developing a family systems approach to rural healthcare: dealing with the 'heavy-user' problem. *Fam Sys Health.* **14**: 291–302.

Larivaara P, Taanila A, Huttunen I, Väisänen E, Moilanen I and Kiuttu J (2000) From biomedical teaching to biopsychosocial education: a process of change in a Finnish medical school. *J Interprof Care.* **14**: 375–85.

Launer J (1995) General practice and primary care: the AFT special interest group. *Context.* **23**: 27–8.

Leff J, Vearnals S, Brewin C *et al.* (2000) The London depression intervention trial: randomised control trial of anti-depressants versus couple therapy in the treatment and maintenance of people living with a partner. Clinical outcome and costs. *Br J Psychiatry.* **177**: 95–100.

McDaniel S, Hepworth J and Doherty W (1992) *Medical Family Therapy*. Basic Books, New York.

McFadyen A (1997) Rapprochement in sight? Post-modern therapy and psychoanalysis. *J Fam Ther*. **19**: 241–62.

McNamee S and Gergen K (eds) (1992) *Therapy as Social Construction*. Sage, London.

Minuchin S and Fishman W (1981) *Family Therapy Techniques*. Harvard University Press, London.

Nichols MP and Schwartz RC (2001) *Family Therapy: concepts and methods* (5e) Allyn and Bacon, London.

Palazzoli Selvini M, Boscolo L, Cecchin G and Prata G (1980) Hypothesising-circularity-neutrality: three guidelines for the conductor of the session. *Fam Proc*. **19**: 3–12.

Papadopoulos R and Byng-Hall J (eds) (1997) *Multiple Voices: narrative in systemic family psychotherapy*. Duckworth, London.

Pocock D (1995) Searching for a better story: harnessing modern and post-modern positions in family therapy. *J Fam Ther*. **17**: 149–73.

Seaburn D, Gawinski B, Harp J, McDaniel S, Waxman D and Shields C (1993). Family systems therapy in a primary care medical setting: the Rochester experience. *J Marital Fam Ther*. **19**: 177–90.

Selvini Palazzoli M, Boscolo L, Cecchin G and Prata G (1978) *Paradox and Counterparadox: a new model in the therapy of the family in schizophrenic transaction*. Jason Aronson, New York.

Senior R (1994) Family therapy in general practice: 'We have a clinic here on a Friday afternoon . . .'. *J Fam Ther*. **16**: 313–27.

Tomson D and Czauderna J (1994) Family therapy and primary care: connections and challenges. *J Fam Ther*. **16**: 342–4.

Tomson P and Asen E (1987) Can GPs be taught family therapy methods? A contribution to the debate. *Fam Sys Med*. **5**: 97–104.

Tomson P (1990) GPs and family therapy: a dialogue. *J Fam Ther*. **12**: 97–104.

Von Bertalanffy L (1968) *General System Theory*. George Braziller, New York.

Watzlawick T, Bavelas JB and Jackson DD (1967) *Pragmatics of Human Communication*. Norton, New York.

White M and Epston D (1990) *Narrative Means to Therapeutic Ends*. Norton, New York.

CHAPTER 11

The training

When we first set about designing a basic training for primary care professionals, we settled on several guidelines (Launer and Lindsey 1997).

- Any training should address the whole range of work with patients, both 'psychological' and 'medical', as well as looking at interactions between professionals.
- It should be presented from a coherent basis of modern social constructionist and narrative approaches.
- It should be taught didactically and also modelled by our questioning of participants and our interaction with each other.
- Our teaching should be based on the fundamental ideas of observation, together with contexts, patterns, processes and beliefs.
- We should introduce participants to the art of asking questions in a way that does not presuppose that doctors or nurses have prior or superior knowledge of what is going on.
- We should encourage a non-interpretative stance, where it is more important to listen to language than to make assumptions about hidden or 'underlying' meanings.
- Our aim should be to map out a field of thought which we believe might support and facilitate primary care, while letting participants see our uncertainty about how these ideas might be useful.

In many ways, the courses that we now teach still echo many of the ideas and themes that we first settled on. This particularly includes an emphasis on contexts, and on the way that contexts determine the meaning of people's stories. However, there has been a considerable evolution in the teaching. We have learned, through trial and error, which ideas transfer well to primary care and which do not. We have had to respond to the emergence of some of the ideas (like 'narrative' itself) from relative obscurity into the common parlance of many practitioners. We have therefore had to find more sophisticated ways of presenting these. In particular, we have had to meet requests from course participants to focus on specific narrative techniques, rather than just the overall framework of thinking.

The following sections give a description of the trainings as we now conduct them.

The courses

The pilot course in 1995 ran for one afternoon a week, for a single ten-week term. It attracted 13 GP participants, two health visitors and one practice nurse. Following this we ran a subsequent course for a new intake, which we extended to a year at the request of most of the participants. In the years since then, we have encouraged everyone whenever possible to follow the course for two or three terms. This allows us to focus on video material brought by students, to show work with actual families through a screen and to include a wider range of reading, including literature from the social sciences concerning medicine, gender and ethnicity. We have come to believe that the benefits of a year's training are far greater than a single term in bringing about far-reaching attitudinal change and skills development.

In addition to the main courses, we have run brief introductory courses in England and Israel lasting from one to four days. As a result of one of these, we helped to set up a continuing study group based in the Department of Postgraduate Family Medicine at the University of Tel Aviv. We have also run workshops in Holland and Finland. In the time we have been doing both the longer and short courses, we have developed a particular approach. The rest of this chapter is a description of this.

Over seven years we have taught about 120 practitioners on our main courses at the Tavistock and several hundred more in shorter events there and elsewhere. We have also had an increasing amount of input into GP vocational training courses, trainers' courses and educational events for other professionals, including community pharmacists and optometrists.

All the courses are taught by people who are family therapists as well as having a core discipline as GP, clinical psychologist, psychiatrist or social worker. Nearly all the teachers have had some direct experience of working in primary care settings as clinicians, educators, researchers or consultants.

Philosophy

In accordance with family therapy thinking, we try to design all teaching activities in a way that helps participants 'unlearn' conventional linear thinking by de-emphasising such concepts as simple cause and effect, unitary diagnosis or medical objectivity. This is not to say that we do not respect these concepts where appropriate, but we see our role as being to introduce some significant difference into participants' understanding of how consultations might be conducted. Our exercises are therefore governed by the following emphases:

- interaction more than individuals
- process more than content
- beliefs and values more than objective truths
- multiple perspectives more than single ones
- empowerment more than paternalism
- allowing evolution of narrative rather than problem solving.

Our approach includes some of the traditional techniques used in postgraduate GP education, such as role play or case discussions, while making connections with underlying theory that might help participants to understand why narratives develop as they do. We feel that the use of practical exercises is the best way to give learners an authentic experience of thinking and feeling in terms of an evolutionary rather than a fixed reality, and to develop the ability to hold multiple descriptions in their minds during any consultation. They also give an opportunity to explore practical ways in which narrative thinking and techniques can be brought into almost any interaction with patients and fellow team members.

We have come to think that our work is to some extent reparative. It helps people to undo sometimes years of stereotypical consulting styles which may have been acquired either during the long and arid period of biomedical education or (more depressingly) during a subsequent period of GP vocational training which may have been based too rigidly on one single approach to the consultation, even if that approach might be a more liberal or 'enlightened' one. The activities we use are therefore examples of the practical ways in which we have tried to move course participants from more conventional styles of thinking towards a consideration of how they and their patients might generate more imaginative stories.

Curriculum

For any initial term's teaching, and for short courses, we try to cover the following topics:

- what is narrative thinking?
- conversations inviting change
- the family network: geneograms
- the professional network and personal values
- social and political values and their effects

- narrative approaches to physical illness
- supervision and consultancy.

For any subsequent terms, we concentrate more extensively on developing techniques for narrative-making conversations and for mutual case consultancy. We also go more deeply into some of the dilemmas of a narrative approach to severe physical illness, and we look at ways of integrating narrative thinking with medical, nursing or other primary care work. We also select particular themes for some sessions, including ethnicity, gender and power. According to the wishes of the group, we may address specific areas of interest: these have included asthma, disability, frequent consulters, behaviour problems, child abuse, work with couples, eating disorders, drugs and alcohol, and cancer. We have also taken the opportunity to look for comparison at some other more normative and directive family therapy models, somewhat different from our own, including structural and strategic family therapy, and at the biopsychosocial model.

Theoretical presentations and reading

Unlike many courses addressing consultation skills, we spend between a quarter and a third of any course focusing on theory. We present this either in the form of brief lectures or as set reading. For a ten-week course we would probably set eight or nine published articles with a narrative viewpoint, taken from journals and books from the worlds of family therapy, primary care or social science. Our emphasis on theoretical material arises directly from our experience of therapy training: therapists are always expected to master the intellectual and conceptual framework within which they will be working. From what we have seen, primary care clinicians soon acquire an appetite for reading and even become avid for it. Some have never been asked to read professional material of any intellectual depth since they finished their basic training, and some (including the older nurses) have no prior experience of this at all. Occasional complaints about the reading being impenetrable are vastly outnumbered by expressions of pleasure at being challenged to think about sophisticated abstract ideas.

Apart from pure mental stimulation, another motive we have is to give people a thorough grounding in a theoretical field of major contemporary importance which is unknown to many people from primary care. This demonstrates that we are not lone eccentrics within the wider therapeutic and academic worlds, and also exposes learners to the scale, consistency and cogency of the critique that this field offers to conventional medical ways of thinking and acting. This can be a shock, but it is nearly always an exciting and creative shock.

Teaching exercises

We devote much of any teaching session to exercises involving active participation. Initially on any course we concentrate on role play, but as people acquire greater skill we spend more time on mutual case supervision, in which members of the group take turns to interview each other on cases from their daily work where they are experiencing difficulties. While role play is especially helpful for introducing entirely new skills, its artificiality can limit the level of sophistication involved in the exercise. Mutual supervision requires a higher degree of skill to be effective, but it has the enormous advantage of having immediate efficacy for the clinician who has the chance to be interviewed by a colleague about a troubling case. Most participants say they learn more in the long run from interviewing each other about real cases than by adopting roles, and that any skills learned in this way – particularly those of effective questioning – can be readily transferred to consultations with patients as well. We move between a focus on the individual patient, the couple and the family, and we try to be careful to include cases that focus on non-nuclear families or those of different cultural origins.

The purpose of all these activities is on developing micro-skills for the consultation, and especially on using an exact choice of language in conversing with patients. Our initial preference for this has been strongly reinforced over the years by all our experience. Participants regularly report that their professional and postgraduate trainings have hitherto focused at too global a level of thought or feeling, whereas they find that an emphasis on the precise wording of a response or a question requires learners to concentrate more fully on the effects of their interventions. Paradoxically, we find that concentrating on micro-skills often produces a more substantial change in beliefs and attitudes than previous attempts to influence these in more general ways.

As an example of this, we try to discourage people from psychologising formulations such as '*I think my patient's in denial*'. In common with most narrative thinkers nowadays, we regard such formulations as paternalistic, unhelpful and distancing. Rather than lecturing about this, we prefer to demonstrate, or to elicit from a group, how one might manage a consultation in which the clinician started to have such thoughts. For example, we might suggest that the group discussed:

- '*What questions could you ask to check out whether the patient has a different view of serious illness from your own?*' or
- '*How can you create an opportunity for the patient to express fear and grief without insisting that this is the only correct behaviour?*'

Using the same techniques, it is also easier to help people to move from a preoccupation with the content of problems and to focus instead on processes, values and beliefs. For example, if course members bring cases where they are over-involved or stuck, it is often more helpful for interviewers to ask relatively few questions about the precise details of each case. It may be more useful to ask more about how practitioners view themselves in their jobs, or what responsibilities they believe they have towards their patients. Working together, the observers and tutor can usually help to direct interviewers towards such questions, with more benefit to the interviewees.

Some techniques: observers, 'freeze frame' and the reflecting team

We frequently make use of observers in all our role play and case consultancy practice. Observers notice things about the content and process of conversations that participants cannot, because they are too involved. They can therefore help interviewers by drawing their attention to these. Through watching others, observers also become aware of common errors such as inattention to crucial information or inappropriate timing. Later they can use this awareness to improve their own practice.

We find that the use of observers is particularly powerful in combination with another technique that we call the 'freeze frame', by analogy with the button for freezing a video recording. We give participants the right to 'freeze' a conversation at any stage so that they can come out and have a discussion with the observer or observers. Equally, an observer can ask for the participants to stop so that he or she can make an observation or suggest a hypothesis or question. We encourage interviewers to take such breaks as often as they wish, after every question or response if necessary. In this way we give them permission to put their consulting technique under the microscope in a controlled environment. This can be particularly helpful in the early stages of reorienting themselves to a non-linear approach to the consultations, where beginners commonly 'freeze' their exercises at an early stage to say: *'I know what I'd normally ask, but it isn't very imaginative. Can you please help me think of a better question?'*

We also allow observers the right to freeze any consultation, but we ask them to be sparing in such interventions. It is obviously less disruptive for the interviewer in any exercise to choose the best moment to pull out for reflection rather than being forcibly withdrawn from the conversation by an observer. Also, we want observers to see themselves as a resource for the interviewer, and therefore to make themselves available in ways that the interviewer might find most useful rather than jumping in on their own initiative too often. We are, in effect, creating a concentric system, so the observer is acting as consultant to the interviewer, who is acting as a consultant to the role-play patient or presenting clinician. To put it the other way round, the patient is the client of the interviewer, who in turn is the client of the observer.

Following the usual conventions of family therapy training, we tend to impose a fairly tight set of rules on such exercises. (Readers who are not themselves educators may want to skip the more technical descriptions that take up the rest of this chapter, and move on to the next chapter or the following one.)

- The observer cannot talk directly to the role-play 'patients' or client. This maintains the authority of the interviewer and gives him or her some helpful reflective time away from the heat of the consultation itself.
- The role-play 'patients' or consulting client can listen in to the conversation between their interviewer and the observer, but they cannot join in. This gives them the opportunity to hear alternative stories to the ones being pursued by their interviewer without the consultation becoming confused by several different lines of thought being pursued at the same time.
- When there is one observer only, we sometimes suggest that he or she uses the breaks in the session to *interview* the interviewer, for example, about how the interviewer is finding the consultation so far, what stories are being pursued, etc. Interviewers often say they find this more helpful than simply hearing suggestions. This is hardly surprising, since the whole point of our teaching is to demonstrate that interventive interviewing is more liberating for everyone concerned than trying to solve someone else's problems.
- When there are several observers, we may suggest that each in turn offers a hypothesis, followed by a possible question that might be asked to test that hypothesis. By structuring their comments in this way, observers are less likely to make the interviewer or the clients feel swamped.
- Alternatively, where there are several observers, we may suggest that they have a discussion in front of the role-play 'patients' or client. The interviewer may or may not choose to take a part in this. Thus, the group of observers becomes a reflecting team. When the interviewer returns to conducting the interview, it is often good practice to ask the patients or client: '*Of all the ideas and questions you have heard the team discuss, which has seemed the most helpful?*' The interviewer can then base the next part of the interview on the response.
- As a variant of this, we sometimes use the structure of having an interviewer, a single observer to help the interviewer and a reflecting team to act as back up to the single observer. It can be a useful discipline to have the interviewer listen silently while the observer gets consultancy from the reflecting team.

Although these rules can seem pedantic and even irksome at first, we find that the discipline of following them becomes increasingly helpful. They make the teaching points clearer and are more likely to produce a worthwhile outcome for anyone in the group who is trying to find alternative ideas for an active clinical case. The benefits of bringing out multiple perspectives, testing hypotheses and drawing attention to feedback that might have been missed can provide more than ample justification for an edifice of reflective devices that might otherwise appear quite obsessive.

Security

In relation to role-play exercises, we always tell participants that there is a requirement to avoid confrontation or entertainment since this is usually counterproductive in an educational context. Many exercises of the kind we use have a potential for going out of control if not sensitively handled, so we believe it is also important to do the following.

- *Obtain consent.* Some participants are initially uncomfortable with role play and, if so, we permit them to take just an observing role in the early weeks. (In all such cases, we find they volunteer to engage in role play long before we feel any need to push them into it.) Whenever we design an exercise where personal material is requested we always offer an alternative. For example, participants who do not wish initially to bring their own geneograms for discussion in pairs are told that they are welcome to practise this technique at first by recalling a family or dynasty from a soap opera such as *The Archers* or *Eastenders*. (Again, we find that these precautions are scarcely ever necessary beyond the first couple of weeks, but we believe that offering these options is a form of containment that makes participants feels less pressurised and more comfortable.)
- *Clarity of objectives.* The purpose of some exercises will be to practise a particular skill, such as hypothesising or circular questioning. The focus of others will be on the content of the case material itself. To avoid ambiguity, we always try to make it clear what we are doing and why. It may be necessary, for instance, to explain to someone who is bringing a case for the purpose of an exercise, that they may not be helped with practical solutions for dealing with that case. We are effectively borrowing the case material for an educational rather than a clinical purpose. Occasionally exercises depend for their value on a gradual understanding of their purpose rather than an immediate one. So in some cases, we might not declare all of our hand at the outset, but it is especially important in such instances that we as tutors are very clear in our own minds about our educational objectives.
- *Deroling.* In common with all educators who undertake role-play exercises, we think it is very important for all participants to 'derole' under each exercise. This involves each participant who has taken on an active role saying 'I am not [role just played], my real name is [real name] and in real life I am a

health visitor in ...'. This provides some protection against the possibility of taking away some of the emotional conflicts raised by exercises.

Case discussions

In common with other primary care educators, we find that case discussions can too easily become a free-for-all. The person holding the difficult case is bombarded with suggestions, advice and even criticism. He or she can end up feeling either persecuted or inadequate or both. To prevent this, we try to emphasise the fact that the presenter is in fact a client, and the rest of the group should function as a consulting system. For a consulting system to work well, it needs to be able to operate in much the same way as an interview.

In the early stages of any course, we try to discourage straightforward case discussion altogether, on the grounds that participants have not yet learned the discipline of consulting with each other in a neutral and facilitative way. Some are likely to be stuck within conventional modes of advice giving, particularly in a group context. (Doctors especially seem to find it hard to free themselves from going off on anecdotal tangents with stories that generally begin '*I had a very similar case* ...'.) A minority have acquired a habitual stance of offering 'ex cathedra' psychodynamic or pseudopsychodynamic interpretations of either the patient's or the doctor's behaviour. Once we have taught some basic skills in questioning and interviewing, we use opportunities to have mutual case consultancy in 'fishbowls', with the group as a whole working as a reflecting team. This can be seen as a halfway stage on the road to proper team consultancy, the group now functioning as a resource for developing new narratives and not just a debating society.

When a course group as a whole seems to be working well as a reflecting team, open case discussion becomes a real and effective possibility. Members realise, for example, that even in a large group conversation, it is more helpful to pose a question to the person with a problem than to make a statement. They also realise that it is generally better to offer a hypothesis for the client clinician to chew over rather than to pontificate on the probable diagnosis or imagined 'underlying cause' for what is going on. The group members also now have the discipline to follow feedback, developing their ideas from what the clinician has just said, or from a useful comment by someone else in the group, rather than offering an unconnected idea arising from their own preoccupations.

Video review

If case discussion is potentially undermining for the presenting clinician, review of videotapes of live consultations is even more so. It requires similarly strict protective measures to give presenters confidence and also to be of active professional benefit to them. The rules we have developed for our own courses are the following.

- Before showing the video, presenters have a chance to set the context, explaining as much as they feel the group needs to know about the circumstances of the consultation in order to make sense of the tape.
- The group then has a chance to ask any factual questions about the context, for example: '*Have you ever seen other members of the family?*' or '*Does the patient ever consult with anyone else in the practice?*'
- The presenters say what they would like the group to look out for, and what kind of help they would like the group to give them. In other words, they set a specific task for the group. Sometimes this will be oriented around a technical piece of learning, such as, '*Are there any questions I should be asking in order to make better progress with this person?*' Sometimes it may be much more related to the content of the case, for example '*I don't know if I'm right to go on seeing this person on my own or whether I should refer them to a psychiatrist*'.
- The presenters usually hold the remote control and stop at a point in the tape where they particularly want to invite comments. Alternatively, one of the tutors will hold it and select when to stop the tape, but only with the agreement of the presenter that this is a useful juncture at which to invite discussion.
- We encourage the group to follow the same guidelines as for case discussion, namely to seek to facilitate the work through judicious questioning, or by proposing hypotheses for the presenter to consider, rather than through giving advice and suggestions.
- The presenters always have the last word, saying what they found most helpful from the discussion and why, and saying how they think they might use these ideas in proceeding with the case.

Generally, we have the expectation that the shorter the piece of tape shown, the more productive the work will be. Although groups have an understandable curiosity to see 'how it all ended', the development of precise and effective consulting micro-skills depends much more on presenters being able to reflect on such things as turn of phrase, timing or even intonation. Positive feedback from a presenter often comes in response to something as simple, and as small, as an idea for one possible question that could be asked at the next encounter with the patient in question.

Confidentiality

At the beginning of each course, and repeatedly during them, we emphasise that all material used on the course, whether introduced by us or disclosed by participants, is 'within these four walls only'. In addition, we make it clear that participants may choose to share or not to share material with the group entirely according to their own wishes, whether this relates to their own lives or their encounters with patients. Self-evidently, these ground rules are more important in relation to some exercises than others.

Cost

It is conventional to write about postgraduate teaching methods without mentioning money. Yet educational activities are embedded within political and financial contexts. Their creation, development and success derive from those contexts – and in turn influence them. We do not avoid discussing with course participants some of the issues and dilemmas that surround the financial aspects of the course.

The fee for one term's course (ten half-days) has been over £400. This covers staff time, the use of the Clinic library, overheads and tea. For some professions outside primary care, particularly psychologists and psychotherapists, spending such sums on one's continuing professional development (CPD) is routine. This is not the case within primary care. Except for enthusiasts who go off to study for MAs or particular specialities, GPs are mostly used to having their postgraduate education subsidised by pharmaceutical companies or hospital postgraduate centres. Primary care nurses rarely have sums of this size to spare. Professions like pharmacy, optometry and dentistry have no tradition in Britain of regular CPD, although from time to time they may go on specific courses aimed at enhancing their technical skills and commercial success.

As a result, we have almost never been able to run our courses (except for short ones) solely with fee-paying participants. We have depended to a large degree on linkage with regional or district schemes giving subsidies to people who wanted to attend. For some years, most of the GPs we taught were funded as part of the London Implementation Zone fund for educational initiatives (LIZEI) – a crisis-drive scheme to promote 'recruitment, refreshment and retention' of GPs at a time when their numbers in the city were falling disastrously. When the LIZEI scheme came to an end, there was a hiatus. This meant that for a total of three terms out of the past seven years we have been unable to run courses.

In more recent years, we have cultivated a relationship with our local health authority. They have paid both fees and a locum subsidy for any primary care professional with clinical responsibility who wished to attend. We have therefore developed a valuable local network of people who work within the vicinity of the Clinic and have got to know each other well as a result of studying together. We have also been able to attract far more health visitors, practice nurses and district nurses, as well as welcoming for the first time some pharmacists, optometrists and dentists. At the same time, however, we have had to focus on some topics of immediate current interest to the health authority as commissioners, particularly the transition to primary care groups and trusts (PCGs and PCTs). Although we have continued to attract individual fee-paying students from as far afield as Kent, Bristol and Devon, the courses have to some extent lost their national flavour.

These political realities raise some interesting questions, not just for us and our course members but for people involved in primary care generally. For training like ours to survive and grow, one of two things will need to happen. Either the culture of primary care clinicians will have to change so that people regularly make a personal investment in their own professional development, or statutory bodies like PCTs will need to play a serious role in promoting types of training that aim for long-term attitudinal and skills development.

References

Launer J and Lindsey C (1997) Training for systemic general practice: a new approach from the Tavistock Clinic. *Br J Gen Pract.* 47: 453–6.

CHAPTER 12

Some teaching exercises

This chapter gives some sample exercises in detail. Partly this is to provide a resource for other primary care educators, but it is also a way of demonstrating how a narrative-based approach can be introduced to people who are unfamiliar with it. Versions of some of these exercises have been published previously in the journal *Education for General Practice* (Launer 1996, 1998a, b, 1999a, b, c).

The majority of our exercises involve no more than saying *'get into groups of three and take it in turns – for about 30 minutes each – to be the interviewer, the observer or the person talking about a case that's bothering you'*. We then move around the room and focus on honing people's questioning skills. Alternatively we may ask for someone to present a case related to the topic of the session (children at risk or marital work, for example). We then invite some of the group to role play the family while the others take it in turns as interviewers and members of the reflecting team. For reasons discussed in Chapter 11, we interrupt such exercises very freely. Usually we do this to help either small or large groups consider how a question or other intervention might be formulated to better effect. We may also do it for other reasons, for example to check that the person being interviewed is happy to continue with the exercise.

However, on certain occasions, particularly for illustrating complex issues, we use some quite elaborate exercises including 'semi-scripted role play' (Launer 1996). We do this particularly in the earlier part of courses when we are first introducing people to basic concepts and skills. This chapter covers some of these exercises.

Learning from your own geneogram

One effective way of learning how to balance curiosity with tact, or how to focus quickly on what is important to someone's story, is by drawing and studying your own geneogram – possibly with a colleague who is willing to do the same in return.

Many people initially consider that their own geneograms will prove boring to others, something that is very rarely the case. Familiarity prevents people noticing the uniqueness of their own family story, but exposure to interview by a comparative stranger brings out that uniqueness. Nearly everyone reports that having their geneogram elicited is a moving experience, leading them to make connections they had never previously considered and to gain new understanding of how the past has influenced the present. Some people have been inspired to go on and do some interviews within their own families, either for historical or for personal and reparative reasons.

One thing to consider when doing this is how to prevent it turning into a kind of personal therapy. It is important for people who take each other's geneograms to know they do not have to disclose any information they do not want to, and that they can indicate this to their interviewers. In spite of this, professionals do sometimes want to disclose difficult things in their family past. This has to be handled delicately, but it provides an opportunity to learn the appropriate sensitivity for dealing with similar situations when they arise while taking geneograms from patients.

We ask every course group to spend a session working in pairs on their own geneograms. In primary care consultations, the focus of a geneogram is usually clear: it is an attempt to gain a wider understanding of a problem. Working with colleagues, the focus is less clear so we sometimes offer these suggestions.

- *'Focus on how first names are assigned in the family, and what they mean.'* Most families pay careful attention to the naming of new members, and the choices made by the various generations or branches of a family can yield important meaning, e.g. the transition from biblical to secular names, or a tradition of passing down the names of honoured forebears.
- *'Focus on any differences of ethnicity, religion or social class within the family, and what these differences mean.'* In the most seemingly homogeneous families, small nuances of social or religious difference can take on enormous importance. In reality, most of the families described by any group of professionals in inner London in the early 21st century will reveal an astonishingly rich diversity of origins and identities.
- *'Focus on trying to understand what influences within the family might have led your interviewee to choose their particular career.'* Doctors and nurses may come from families with strong traditions of professional caring, but they may also come from families where illness and suffering has figured importantly, or where medical and nursing training has signified particular virtues or kinds of social achievement.

Normative and narrative interviewing

Primary care professionals are generally schooled in a kind of interviewing that assumes that medical reality is the normative one against which the patient's experiences must be measured. This exercise gives people a chance to explore the possibilities and limits of taking a narrative-based approach.

The structure is very simple. We divide the large group into threes or fours: each small group then chooses a presenter, an interviewer and one or two observers. We ask each presenter to think of one particular patient who has an unconventional view of their own medical condition (in terms of its nature, its cause or the treatment needed). The presenter in each small group then has a chance to describe that patient briefly.

We then ask the presenters to 'turn themselves into the patient' and take on that person's role for a consultation. We ask the interviewers to run the consultation twice over – allowing 10 to 15 minutes each time. The first time, we suggest that interviewers should hold on to their normal consulting style. While being reasonably tolerant of the patient's unorthodox beliefs, they should continue to act on the basis that their own medical view of the complaint is 'normative' and has absolute authority. Within the limits of normal courtesy, they should try to persuade the patient of the 'reality' of their diagnosis and the reasons for recommending treatment.

For the second performance of the consultation, however, we ask interviewers to act as if they are anthropologists. We invite them to try and enter the patient's conceptual world without any prejudice or assumptions, regarding what is and is not an acceptable description of reality.

The following issues usually emerge from this exercise.

- *It is very difficult to stay neutral.* Even the most accomplished practitioners are surprised how hard it is to sustain a genuinely inquisitive and uncritical stance, especially when faced with beliefs or behaviour that appear to fly in the face of conventional medical wisdom. For most doctors and nurses, knowledge of what is scientifically 'true' is so deeply ingrained that they will constantly display their professional mind-set, in spite of their very best efforts.
- *Patients are uncomfortable with total neutrality.* One common finding in this exercise is that the 'patients' find it impossible to *allow* their interviewers to remain neutral. Their own expectations of healthcare professionals are so inflexible that they anticipate that their views will be opposed, and therefore exert pressure on their interviewers to take an oppositional stance. When the interviewers do succeed in expressing permissiveness towards their beliefs, the 'patients' may become quite disconcerted. This demonstrates how patients may need professionals to remain within their expected social roles rather than try to 'get out of the frame' through an excess of empathy.
- *Neutrality causes dilemmas.* Interviewers who genuinely try to demonstrate neutrality in this exercise can encounter some quite acute dilemmas. For example, they may find themselves becoming drawn into a collusive agreement with any ideas that are dangerous or delusional (for example, if their

patient says: '*Vitamin B12 won't cure my pernicious anaemia, it will only poison me*'). They may also have to grapple with the consequences of listening to a highly partisan view of the world without opposing it ('*All surgeons are killers – they're only in it for the money*'). Direct confrontation of such views will almost certainly fail. On the other hand, total permissiveness towards the patient will completely paralyse the consultation.

This experience compels the group to examine the kinds of difficulty that may arise in real life with patients whose views are at variance with the professional. What the exercise invites people to discover, therefore, is how to show respectful curiosity while still remaining able to describe – but not prescribe – a professional perspective.

Whose agenda is it anyway?

One of our favourite role-play exercises is also probably the most effective one for capturing the interactional nature of primary care consultations. It is focused on the needs of GPs, and requires participants to become aware of the different realities that the patient and the professional can bring.

We start with three sets of instructions. A third of the group are given 'the practitioner's instructions', a third are given 'the patient's instructions' and the remainder given 'the observer's instructions'.

The practitioner's instructions

A 50-year-old patient came to see you two weeks ago with a history that seemed likely to be of angina of recent onset. The patient smokes heavily and weighs 15 stone. Examination showed a BP of 172/108. You asked the patient to see the practice nurse twice in the following week for BP measurement: this was 168/104 and 178/106.

You also asked the patient to have some tests. The results arrived yesterday. ECG shows ischaemic changes. Fasting lipids show moderately raised cholesterol. The other tests are fine.

In a few minutes you are going to see the patient again to explain the results and discuss the diagnosis. How are you going to deal with this and what are your priorities for this consultation?

The patient's instructions

You are 50. You saw your GP two weeks ago. You explained that you have been getting some chest pain recently when walking any distance.

The doctor asked you some questions, examined you, ordered some tests and told you to see the practice nurse a couple of times as your blood pressure seemed high.

Today you are coming back for the results of all the tests. You are quite frightened. Last year your favourite uncle died suddenly from a heart attack. You are worried there is something badly wrong with your heart.

You are overweight and you smoke, but life is stressful and you hate it when doctors go on about this. (Feel free to invent some more biographical background in advance if you wish.)

As a patient, what are your priorities for this consultation? What would you like to get out of it?

The observer's instructions

You are about to watch a consultation between a doctor and a patient. The patient has been suffering from chest pain and is worried. The doctor has ordered some tests which point towards a diagnosis of angina and is going to tell the patient the results.

What do you think the doctor's agenda is likely to be? What do you think the patient's agenda is likely to be? In observing the interaction between practitioner and patient, what do you think it will be interesting to look out for?

Obviously, no group is aware of what appears on the other two groups' instructions. The structure of the teaching session is as follows.

- Each of the three peer groups – practitioners, patients, observers – convenes to discuss the question on their instructions for 10–15 minutes.
- Participants are redistributed into role-play consultations for 10–15 minutes. Each consultation has one practitioner, one patient and one observer. (For this exercise, there is no time for reflective breaks.)
- The three peer groups then reconvene to share their experiences.
- We hold a plenary discussion.

The tensions set up between different kinds of reality in this exercise are acute, but they are also realistic. Increasingly, GPs are held to highly programmatised agendas in the consultation, driven by considerations from the world of population health and preventive medicine (Davies 1984; Toon 1995). At the same time, patients bring highly personal concerns and beliefs, which doctors are also exhorted to pay attention to. The exercise brings these two worlds into stark apposition and therefore challenges those in the doctor's role to make extraordinarily difficult (but not unrealistic) decisions about balancing two quite different types of professional imperative. The typical time constraints of a GP consultation, which we exactly reproduce for this exercise, tighten the screw as they do in the GP's everyday life.

We have conducted this exercise many dozens of times now, both at the Tavistock and elsewhere. In the plenary discussions that we always allow at the end, there has been a range of feedback.

Patients very often report that they feel pressurised or overwhelmed, and that their stories have been ignored. They have encountered doctors during the exercise who have been entirely organised in their thinking by what can be counted, measured or provably prevented, and as a result have shown insensitivity to the patient's own particular anxieties and preferences. A minority of patients, however, say that they have been impressed by their role-play doctor's willingness to tailor information and advice to their own individual circumstances, or to pace this in accordance with their needs to present and develop their own narratives.

Doctors usually say they find the task daunting and frustrating. Following the initial discussion with their peers, they have entered the consultation with a clear set of priorities and a strategy based on the objective 'facts' of the case. This is blown sky high by the patient's level of anxiety, choice of lifestyle or wish to tell a personal story. Many doctors realise afterwards that the patient's agenda has in fact deflected them from offering obvious and simple clinical action, for example advising the patient to start to take aspirin daily – or indeed from making the urgent cardiology referral that seems to be called for here. Most experience serious difficulties with time management, especially with closing the consultation.

Observers are generally struck by the apparent incompatibility of the doctor's various duties – as sympathetic witness, clinical decision maker and practical epidemiologist. They notice how most of the role-play doctors opt for the second and third of these duties, finding it hard to integrate any therapeutic input into this consultation beyond the level of some seemingly impatient counselling-type noises. They often report becoming aware of how evident the doctor's power is in this situation, especially the power of choosing the route for the consultation to take, and for imposing that choice without checking with the patient that this fits in any way with theirs.

It is easy to see this exercise merely as one about developing 'consultation skills', but for us and hopefully those we teach, it is intended to be something wider. It is an example of the enormous number of contexts that govern so many primary care encounters: contexts that are personal, biomedical, statutory, cultural, political, financial and structural. It is meant to bring learners starkly up against the fact that it is simply impossible to negotiate and manage all these contexts together. However, they can be addressed reflectively in pre-consultation discussions with peers and one can strategise the consultation intelligently in collaboration with patients to create a shared narrative. Indeed, the exercise is so structured that it is impossible to have any encounter except a thoroughly unsatisfactory one unless some kind of conversation takes place in which the range of possible priorities is collaboratively examined and then agreed. For this reason, we try whenever possible to allow participants a rerun of the consultation following the plenary discussion. This often results in far more creative consultations. For instance, the doctor is able to make heard the imperative for urgent action on some fronts (hospital referral and aspirin), while allowing the patient to express both fear and a reluctance to make any lifestyle changes at this moment.

Clashing motivations

The next exercise is similar but allows participants to focus on a quite different set of ideas. It is designed for a multidisciplinary group involving practice nurses, health visitors and community pharmacists as well as GPs. A small number of people from the whole group are asked to volunteer as teenage patients and their parents, while almost everyone else in the group divides into 'primary healthcare teams', each containing at least one GP, one practice nurse or health visitor, and an on-site pharmacist. A few remaining people act as observers. All the 'patients and parents' are given one set of instructions, the health professionals are given another and the observers a third.

Instructions for patients and their parents

The family in this role play are a parent and a child aged 14 who has had asthma for about ten years. The teenager has always used salbutamol inhalers 'on demand' and gets through about one a week.

Doctor and nurses at your local surgery have mentioned steroid inhalers before but neither of you are keen on the idea. You have heard that steroids cause unpleasant side effects. There is a child next door whose parents say had to come off steroid inhalers because her bones were not growing properly.

You are about to visit the surgery for a regular six-monthly review, which involves seeing the GP then a nurse or health visitor. If there is a prescription, you will take it to the on-site pharmacist at the surgery. Personally, the teenager does not think the surgery visit is necessary as he/she feels the asthma is pretty stable. However, the teenager has had a bad sore throat for three days and wants to use the opportunity to ask for some antibiotics.

Discuss in your group of 'parents and patients' how you would like the surgery visit to go.

Instructions for the health professionals

As you know, there is a lot of evidence that asthmatic patients do better on inhaled steroids like beclomethasone than 'relievers' like salbutamol. Many patients who use steroid inhalers regularly do not need so many relievers.

The family in this role play are a parent and a 14-year-old child with asthma who does not use inhaled steroids, and usually gets through three or four salbutamol inhalers a month. The teenager's peak flow is generally about 40% below normal. Today, the parent and child are going to come for a regular asthma review at the surgery, which usually involves seeing (in order) a doctor, then a nurse/health visitor. They will then go to take any prescription to the on-site pharmacist.

Note: The local primary care trust is putting pressure on practices to encourage patients to use steroid inhalers. If a practice can reduce prescribing of relievers by 25% during the year it will gain a practice bonus of £3550. There are no rewards for just prescribing more steroid inhalers. Most practices have decided this makes good clinical and financial sense and have also asked their nurses to help them achieve the change.

Discuss in your professional group how best to deal with the family.

Instructions for observers

You are about to watch a series of two consultations: the first by a GP and the second by a nurse/health visitor. The patient is a 14-year-old with asthma, accompanied by a parent. The professionals all want to encourage the use of steroid inhalers. The patient and parent are not keen.

What beliefs do you think the professionals and patient are each likely to have? What will it be interesting to look out for in these conversations? Discuss these questions in your observers group.

The structure for this exercise is as follows.

- Peer group meetings for:
  (a) patients and their parents
  (b) each 'primary healthcare team' (PHCT) and
  (c) observers.
- Each 'family' then attends a series of ten-minute consultations: first with the GP, then with the practice nurse or health visitor, and finally with the pharmacist who dispenses the prescription. (During each professional consultation, we allow the other professionals from that PHCT to watch, along with the formally nominated observers.)
- Further peer group meetings to discuss the experiences.
- A plenary discussion.

This is an immensely rich and productive exercise in terms of the issues and dilemmas it throws up. Some of the recurrent topics of the final plenary discussion are as follows.

Adolescents and their families are not easy to deal with in the consultation. Most primary care clinicians have had no proper training in talking either to teenagers alone in the room or to parents and their children together. Many feel acutely uncomfortable in doing so, especially when there is tension or disagreement in the room, as is so often the case. Quite apart from the peculiar difficulties that have intentionally been built into this role-play scenario, many participants report feeling at a disadvantage simply by virtue of the age of the patient identified here and the presence of the family in the room.

Steroids and antibiotics are examples of treatments that evoke very strong and polarised ideas and feelings on the part of professionals and the public. Conversations around these treatments very often become adversarial, with clinicians finding it difficult to balance the task of eliciting patients' beliefs with the equally important task of 'selling' the best evidence-based treatment (or declining to prescribe in the absence of good evidence). Matters are complicated by the fact that health professionals often have a range of views about the permissibility of prescribing the 'wrong' treatment in order to build an alliance with a family. They may even have personal feelings about certain treatments such as steroids, perhaps based on direct family experience, that go against the consensus of their professional world. There is also an uncomfortable discordance between certain folk beliefs (such as the danger of all steroids) and the professional beliefs from which these originally derived.

Primary healthcare teams are not unproblematic institutions. Although often presented in professional and political literature as a kind of panacea for the public health, they are in practice fraught with role confusion, so that the patient's combined experience of encountering a number of different members can be very confusing. For example, different disciplines may take a different 'party line' about the importance of transferring from beta-agonist to local steroid sprays for asthma, or have quite different views about the nature of monitoring the illness. This role-play exercise has sometimes highlighted the fact that experienced clinicians may be unclear about the skills, knowledge and duties of other disciplines with which they may have worked 'closely' for their entire careers. With the exception of pharmacists themselves, for instance, everyone else seems amazed by the precise, hands-on clinical role that pharmacists undertake. GPs and nurses doing the exercise have been humbled to see that it was often the pharmacist who managed the exquisite tensions of this scenario with the most efficacy and tact.

Financial incentives and disincentives to prescribe are a minefield. This element of the exercise has given rise to some of the most explosive exchanges we have seen in the course of our teaching. Members of one group erupted into cries of '*bastards!*' when they discovered that they had been in the hands of a PHCT that had not seen fit to declare the financial benefit attached to their change of prescribing. However, other learning groups have found this entirely unproblematical, with the doctors arguing that they would have made the change to steroids regardless of any bonus, while the families and observers have said they would not feel aggrieved if their doctors and nurses did well financially as a result. What this emphasises is that there are huge differences among health professionals concerning issues of professional disclosure. Some people see it as an ethical imperative to declare any such interest to patients, while others take a more paternalistic line in arrogating to themselves the decision about what should and should not be disclosed.

Interviewing a couple

Not surprisingly, people coming on our courses rightly expect some skills training in interviewing couples and families. Although we reiterate that we do not offer family therapy training and that the focus of our courses is entirely on everyday primary care in all its dimensions, there would clearly be no point in wilfully avoiding any training in relation to marital and family difficulties. Here is a role-play exercise designed to develop skills in this area.

In this exercise, we divide people into a number of small groups, each of which will appoint two people to act as a married couple, while the rest act as interviewer and observers. The actors are given the following scenario.

> Mr and Mrs B are in their fifties. He is employed full time and she has an afternoon job. They have two teenage children. Mrs B's father died two years ago, but the other three grandparents are alive. Mrs B often sees the doctor with physical problems – none serious. Mr B almost never sees the doctor. Since Christmas Mrs B has had panics every morning. She clings on to Mr B and cries to prevent him leaving. They have decided to come to the doctor

about this. Mr B feels this is a medical problem and hopes the doctor will prescribe pills. Mrs B often complains to her husband that she feels little emotional support from him these days, especially since her father died, and because he has such demanding work. Discuss this for five minutes, building a few extra factors on to the story before you see the doctor.

The interviewer and observers in each of the small groups then receive their instructions.

Mr and Mrs B are in their fifties. He is employed full time and she has an afternoon job. They have two teenage children. Mrs B's father died two years ago, but the other three grandparents are alive. Mrs B often sees the doctor with physical problems – none serious. Mr B almost never sees the doctor. Today Mrs B has booked another appointment. You have noticed that her husband is sitting with her in the waiting room, which has never happened before. Discuss this for five minutes, exploring the ideas you might have as you fetch the couple into your room.

The structure of the exercise is as follows:

- 15 minutes for the couples and the teams to prepare
- 30 minutes for the interview, with the interviewer, observer and reflecting team conferring as described in the previous chapter
- 30 minutes of plenary discussion concerning the pragmatic and clinical points raised.

This exercise raises a multiplicity of issues. Some are technical and relate to the difficulties people experience in conducting marital or family interviews in primary care. Others are more profoundly conceptual, addressing such things as the nature of panics and what sense can be made out of two conflicting, and perhaps incompatible, beliefs about a mental problem.

Technical issues. Exercises like this expose how little training primary care professionals receive either in focusing simultaneously on more than one patient in the family at any time or on dealing with marital differences or conflict in particular. People playing the role of doctor here at first seem to have difficulty in eliciting the two different stories of reality that husband and wife present. The role-play doctors seem to struggle between two equally unacceptable positions. One is to treat the wife as the 'real patient', implicitly siding with her husband's view of matters. The other is to treat the husband as 'the real problem', and consequently to pathologise and alienate a man who genuinely believes he has come along to the surgery to help the doctor understand and treat his wife properly.

Even though presentations like this one must occur regularly in very many surgeries and clinics, many professionals seem ill-equipped to adopt a neutral or curious stance. They find it hard to take both points of view on board so that the couple are helped to reach an understanding of each others' somewhat incomplete story of how things got to be as they are. The exercise therefore provides an opportunity to learn the rudiments of a questioning approach where the interviewer floats non-commitally between opposing positions and tries to facilitate an agreed story rather than feeling obliged to adjudicate and then to reach a 'solution' based on that adjudication.

Conceptual issues. Underlying these technical issues are some important conceptual ones. There is, for example, the question of what constitutes mental illness and what determines it. Is it legitimate, for instance, to regard Mrs B's condition as an illness when (in her view at any rate) it seems so closely connected with her family circumstances? Equally, is it fair to disqualify Mr B's view of her symptoms simply on the grounds that it is now rather unfashionable, except among some psychiatrists, to see mental symptoms in the way he does? It is tempting for course participants to divide along ideological grounds as pro-psychiatry and anti-psychiatry, but a truly neutral stance involves assigning value to either view. The problem for Mr and Mrs B is not whether one of these theoretical positions will eventually prevail in the medical community, but how they are to live with each other while each places a different but socially acceptable construction on their experience.

One dimension of their different constructions, of course, is a gender one. Mrs B's feeling that her problems are related to her personal context and Mr B's characterisation of them as an intrusive pathology are conventionally gendered beliefs. Again, it may be tempting for people doing the exercise to choose positions based on their own gender or their beliefs about gender. This does not necessarily mean that men will side with Mr B while women side with Mrs B. On the contrary, the kind of liberal-minded men who attend Tavistock Clinic courses are more likely to sympathise with Mrs B. Some of the women may be impatient with her over-dependence. Our task, therefore, is to facilitate a new kind of neutrality and curiosity where no value judgements are attached to beliefs and behaviour of any kind. This in turn provokes enquiries about when it is right or wrong to 'adopt a position'. This question itself does not have any easy answers, but it does at least open up a conversation at a more sophisticated level about the boundaries between one's professional and personal identities, and the difference between the interviewer's external task and his or her internal moral position.

Dealing with suspected child abuse

This exercise addresses one of the most difficult areas that GPs and practice nurses might encounter. The scenario, given to all participants, is as follows.

A couple (Mr and Mrs K) have recently come on to the list of Dr A. They are Irish, married, in their late thirties. They have a six-week-old boy called Jeremy, their first child.

A week ago Dr A saw Mrs K and Jeremy for the first time, without an appointment. She brought the baby because of slight feeding difficulties. The baby was fine medically and the doctor reassured Mrs K.

Two days later Mr and Mrs K brought Jeremy again, also without an appointment, because of a bruise under his left eye. The parents had no idea why it was there. They were seen by another partner, Dr B, who arranged for a hospital admission for assessment. The paediatricians kept the family overnight. They came to the conclusion that the parents had handled the child roughly through inexperience but had not intentionally harmed him. They arranged for regular visits from the health visitor. The health visitor has seen them three times and the meetings have gone well.

Yesterday Mr and Mrs K came once more to Dr A, without an appointment, because Jeremy had had diarrhoea on and off for three days. On examination he was not dehydrated but he was a bit floppy and Dr A felt 'something wasn't quite right'. Dr A recommended another paediatric assessment. The parents refused, saying they were too upset last time. They also said they were not prepared to see Dr B again. Dr A gave some Dioralyte.

Today they are due to come for a booked appointment for review. They have brought the baby who is gurgling happily in the waiting room and clearly much better.

Think yourself into your assigned role (as Mr K, Mrs K or Dr A). What do you want to achieve from this consultation? What are your dilemmas? What are you afraid will happen?

The structure of the exercise is as follows.

- Two people need to volunteer as Mr and Mrs K, and one as Dr A.
- The couple go aside for 15 minutes to get into role (which may mean inventing some extra biographical details as well).
- While the Ks are getting into role, the rest of the groups spend their 15 minutes helping Dr A think about how to strategise this consultation. They also appoint an observer, with everyone else becoming a reflecting team.
- Twenty to 30 minutes for the consultation itself, with Dr A being able to ask for a 'freeze frame' break to consult with the observer and/or the whole reflecting team.
- A plenary discussion.

One of the most challenging and also the most shocking things about primary care, and general practice in particular, is that everything can be so phenomenally complicated. In this case, we are caught up in a maelstrom of uncertainty and conflict at so many levels, in a clinical area where everyone has strong feelings and where no one ever feels entirely adequate. All participants in this exercise are agreed on one thing: it captures exactly the uncomfortable, messy, maze-like quality that so often characterises the work itself. Unpacking some of the difficulties that people address when doing this exercise, we usually end up looking at the following issues.

Non-accidental injury. Here there is a possible non-accidental injury that, so far as we are aware, has never been named, let alone proved or disproved. How is Dr A to deal with this best? Is it a prerequisite of any sensible conversation that this now has to be brought into the open, with an inquiry as to how Mr and Mrs K experienced the false accusation (and possibly an undeserved exoneration)? What are the risks of pursuing this with the couple, or of not pursuing it? Three conceptual landmarks seem to help groups that are struggling with these questions. One is a universal agreement that baby Jeremy's needs must come first in determining any working strategy with this family. Second is an idea from the Australian family therapist Michael White (White 1986). He suggests that it is both possible and necessary to keep holding on to a 'double description' of any ambiguous presentation like Jeremy's bruise; this enables one to continue working with this family even though the likelihood is that one may never attain certainty about their guilt or innocence. The third idea comes from the Great Ormond Street child psychiatrist Danya Glaser (Glaser 1991), who argues that it is possible to work with child abusers from a pragmatic position of neutrality without letting go of a strongly held personal moral position of abhorrence or a statutory stance of vigilance.

Ethnicity. To make this case more complex but also more realistic and challenging, we sometimes gave the family in the scenario a clear ethnic identity by assigning them the surname Kilkenny. It is interesting to see how participants in the exercise respond to this, with expressed or unexpressed assumptions that Irish families, for example, are more or less likely to perpetrate abuse. To those who claim that the family's name does not lead them to make assumptions of any kind, we enquire what difference it would make if we had given them an alternative and equally obvious ethnic or class identity (Patel, Cohen, Churchill, Okolo, Wong, etc.). It is hard to resist the inference that it is impossible to practise without prejudice. In common with many family therapists, that is exactly what we would argue (Cecchin *et al.* 1994). The issue therefore becomes one of identifying and analysing how one's own ethnic context and the patient's might be influencing the interaction and, to counterbalance that, considering what alternative constructions might be put on the situation other than those one might automatically assume.

Interprofessional disputes. In this case, there seems to be an implicit disagreement (and an implicit lack of communication) between a GP, a paediatrician and a health visitor. This possibility is certainly sufficient to leave many people who do this exercise feeling that the paediatrician and health visitor may be naive or avoidant of conflict. Among Dr A's tasks is the delicate work with the

K family itself, trying to sustain an alliance with them without being drawn into collusiveness. Yet it seems at least possible that two other professionals have become collusive with them, and Dr A may have to do some therapy within the professional network. One of the things the group has to consider is how he might approach the paediatrician, and the ways in which it is possible, although never easy, for GPs to assert their authority and wisdom in the face of specialist certainty. What difference will it make to Jeremy's safety if Dr A succeeds in doing so, and what are the risks to the baby if Dr A fails in his mission of interprofessional diplomacy?

Rights and responsibilities: hospitals, practices and patients. Every time we have done this exercise, one of the thorniest difficulties to manage centres around the Ks refusal to return to the hospital or to see Dr B again. Although all clinical urgency has vanished, there is now an unhappy precedent for refusing appropriate medical care for a baby. Although this can be read as an understandable emotional reaction to unwarranted suspicions, it is equally likely to presage a saga of worrying and intemperate encounters between the family and the medical profession. The group has to help Dr A make a number of decisions about boundaries and about timing. Supposing the family are asked to find another GP – perhaps because there is a policy that patients must be willing to see any partner, at least in an emergency, or because the practice dare not risk the consequences of a refusal to attend hospital. Is there then a chance that they are being unfairly victimised, or alternatively that Jeremy will one day suffer a serious injury without any health agency being aware that he exists and is vulnerable? How can Dr A manage such imponderables in the consultation with the Ks in a way that at least minimises the risk of the worst kinds of outcome?

Doing the exercise itself, and conducting the discussion afterwards, we make no pretence of having definitive answers to these questions. Rather, what we hope to do is to help clinicians analyse the multiple contexts in which these tremendously hard cases are embedded. We also aim to help them to make informed decisions about practical strategies; to operationalise these strategies with thoughtful interventions based on sophisticated micro-skills; and to try and create a space for the family and the carers to create a new and more harmonious story.

References

Cecchin G, Lane G and Ray W (1994) *The Cybernetics of Prejudices in the Practice of Psychotherapy.* Karnac, London.

Davies C (1984) General practitioners and the pull of prevention. *Soc Health Illn.* **6**: 267–89.

Glaser D (1991) Neutrality and child abuse: a useful juxtaposition? *Hum Sys.* **2**: 149–60.

Launer J (1996) Semi-scripted role play: a teaching technique for exploring clinical and ethical dilemmas in GP consultations. *Educ Gen Pract.* **7**: 353–5.

Launer J (1998a) Teaching systemic general practice: a guide to conducting group exercises. I: General principles for group exercises. *Educ Gen Pract.* **9**: 344–7.

Launer J (1998b) Teaching systemic general practice: a guide to conducting group exercises. II: Some basic exercises. *Educ Gen Pract.* **9**: 441–3.

Launer J (1999a) Teaching systemic general practice: a guide to conducting group exercises. III: Developing interview skills. *Educ Gen Pract.* **10**: 72–5.

Launer J (1999b) Teaching systemic general practice: a guide to conducting group exercises. IV: Using supervisors and teams. *Educ Gen Pract.* **10**: 176–9.

Launer J (1999c) Teaching systemic general practice: a guide to conducting group exercises. V: Developing skills for complex problems. *Educ Gen Pract.* **10**: 282–93.

Toon P (1995) Health checks in general practice. *BMJ.* **310**: 1083–4.

White M (1986) Negative Explanation, Restraint and Double Description: a template for family process. *Fam Proc.* **25**: 169–84.

CHAPTER 13

The effects of narrative-based training

Since we first developed a training for primary care, we have sought information about its effects. As each course progresses, we hear from participants about their attempts to incorporate new ideas into their work, and about their successes and failures. We also give regular opportunities for learners to put their thoughts into writing, in the form of semi-structured questionnaires at the halfway and final points of every term, and in an extended essay at the end of a year.

Some of the feedback we elicit is for our own purposes as teachers. For example, we want to know about our own strengths and weaknesses as educators, the impact made by invited tutors, the usefulness of the various exercises or set reading we present, and about the selection of the concepts, techniques or topics that make up our curriculum. We also ask course people to score the educational style and content of their course on a numerical scale. The average scores are generally high, and are useful for internal and external audit. However, our main concern is with the general personal and professional effects of the learning. To find out about this, we regularly ask course participants for written and anonymous responses to questions like these:

- What aspects of the course have you found most helpful/most challenging/ most enjoyable so far?
- What worked least well for you? What would you recommend we do differently?
- In what way has your thinking changed?
- In what way has your practice changed?
- What would you say your work setting's view of this training has been?
- How do you think that you have managed being a trainee while holding on to your competence as a professional in your setting?
- Are there ways in which you look at things differently because of the course? If so, how?

- Are there things you are coping with better because of the course? If so, what?
- What difficulties have you encountered in trying to apply your learning?
- Has the course influenced the way you function in your team and practice? If so, how?
- Any other comments?

This chapter reports on the responses to these questions over the past seven years. The responses have been selected through thematic analysis, by looking at the themes that occur most commonly, and by quoting from passages that encapsulate these.

The comments given here are only a brief selection of many years' feedback, but they are representative. In terms of educational research, they are only a beginning. They report only on learners' reactions, without an external appraisal of their learning, their behaviour or their impact on patients (Kirkpatrick 1967; Kiuttu *et al.* 1996). The resources needed for higher level evaluations are hard to find, and reliable measures for such research are lacking (Hutchinson 1999). Nevertheless, these comments stand as a narrative of their own, and accord in a number of ways with current educational thinking. They are presented here with a minimum of discussion, so that readers can form their own impressions of the feedback – warts and all.

General effects

On every course, the commonest remarks usually concern the area of general professional revitalisation:

> I have regained some enthusiasm for my job. I feel validated in the difficulties I have. I understand more of the system I am part of. I have stopped being too responsible.

> I can bring about change without being bogged down.

> I am thinking about my thinking processes.

> My thinking has changed radically, created a sense of options being available when a personal system is stuck.

> I feel more equal to my male partner.

> I know my limits and capabilities better.

> Objectivity/curiosity has liberated me from the role of problem solver: Doctor fixit.

Here is one longer comment on the theme of general change:

> I have changed the way I perceive myself as a doctor and the context of my work. Using a social constructionist view, I no longer 'know' that I am 'right' about either diagnoses or treatments as I have learned to look beyond the medical model through the gaze of social constructionism. In one sense, medical 'reality' has ceased to exist for me. As a GP, I had already learned to ride several horses at once, for example making diagnoses in the physical, psychological and social frames. From learning something of social constructionism, I feel that I have learned also to ride a chimera. This is both exciting, and rather uncomfortable.

Coupled with this sense of a general change in their work, people also report receiving academic and intellectual stimulation:

> I appreciated the contact with academics and . . . the impetus to read some fairly difficult papers.

> It has been very enjoyable to participate in a course where any reading is required.

Others, however, have particularly noted the provisional nature of the ideas we offer:

> I think you are still developing your thoughts . . . I don't think you feel it is a fixed process yet. I would like to know how you would put it in a few years' time.

Mutual support

Our courses are not designed with the primary aim of setting up a multi-professional peer support group. Nevertheless, course participants are often struck by this more than anything else:

> I enjoyed working in a multidisciplinary group very much and the company of the group was much appreciated.

> Interaction with other healthcare professionals – interesting how situations are tackled from different angles.

> I learned a lot from group work and listening to real-life situations that other participants are coming across.

I realise that other healthcare professionals do not always see that a provision of a prescription for medication is necessarily the outcome of every situation. As a pharmacist I used to think that was the case.

Acquiring skills

Most course participants have come to course sessions straight from work each week. Nearly all have been engaged in demanding clinical jobs. Feedback has most often emphasised how the course has helped to equip them with new skills for dealing with everyday consultations:

> I have managed to listen to my consultations again and feel I can ask different questions.

> Recognise just how prescriptive I am in most consultations.

> Much better at recognising boundaries – in particular avoiding over-engagement. Don't feel stuck with patients to anywhere near the same extent.

> Generating solutions from interventive interviewing rather than prescribing them.

> I have become more questioning and analytical and become more open to not pigeon-holing patients as 'difficult', 'heart sink' etc.

> I ask many more questions about the family. I value patients' stories, ideas about their illness more. I invite relatives to attend too (with less terror).

> Surprisingly, patients don't seem to think anything is odd or inappropriate – so far as I can tell, that is.

One student commented how we model a particular approach by our method of teaching:

> I admired how the tutors coped with attitudes which to me sometimes seemed to be ignorant and how they used these attitudes of people in a situation to demonstrate the communication skills we were supposed to learn. Through the tutor's tolerance to see always the positive aspect in the remark or question I felt very supported.

Here is a longer comments on the theme of skills:

> I would say that the most important change which has relaxed my consulta-
> tion style has come from the idea of asking questions and then asking more
> questions, rather than reaching for statements and facts. It has been a diffi-
> cult discipline to learn, in the face of patients wanting a polished 'expert
> medical answer' to a problem. Keeping the questioning and hypothesising
> pores open is almost a physical, as well as an intellectual, discipline, as it
> embodies the doctor's posture and non-verbal communication to a great
> degree. It says 'let's think about this together' rather than 'you are the
> supplicant and I am the oracle ...'. It goes without saying, of course, that
> vigilance, scanning for serious illness – whether mental or physical, and
> the medical skills which I have alluded to play as full a role as they ever
> did. I have found that, in patients with life-threatening or terminal illness,
> I am placing them in the context of their families more than I used to.

One student offered the following thoughts regarding her listening skills:

> I always felt I was a good listener. I feel that I have changed the quality and
> depth of my listening skills. I listen not just to the story or conversation but
> also to the meaning of what is being said. I am also starting to hypothesise
> why the patient has chosen to talk about a particular situation/person.
> I throw my thoughts back to the patient, making links, sometimes 'good'
> links' sometimes 'not so good', including the social context. I offer the ana-
> logy of knitting a piece of cloth, which becomes rich in texture as the social
> context is explored. My using some of the circular questions in this two-
> way conversation becomes more focused in less time.

Obstacles to learning

Feedback in the area of skills can also be mixed. People have reported frankly on
the difficulties that prevent them using these skills:

> I feel frustrated at work by being aware of a skill which could energise my
> work, but not being sufficiently skilled yet.

> Struggling out of the familiar cocoon of ten years individually orientated
> practice.

> My consultations are longer, list is growing and I am exhausted ...
> early days.

> Whatever we learned is very difficult to implement in practice and daily life.

> As the course is 'deskilling' initially it can be a bit demoralising.

> I leave the course full of ideas of how to use this in practice and with which
> patients. I still have a big leap to make in putting it into practice.

> It has become more chaotic as I try out some of the ideas.

> I think that I will come back to this work later on – but to take it further at
> present would have too destabilising an effect.

> Perhaps I have not changed that much as yet, or do we just resume our hat
> in a surgery setting?

The following longer comment strikes a fairly typical balance between a sense of
achievement and a sense of having incompletely mastered the skills:

> By slowly understanding the principles and general ideas of family ther-
> apy – circularity, context and curiosity – interactions in my professional
> life as well as in my personal life gained a new dimension. I felt from the
> middle of the course relieved because I learned to see problems in a different
> way. I learned to rephrase my questions in order to overcome stuckness,
> frustration and gaps .... Although I feel that asking the right questions in
> a situation is very much an art and I still think for myself, it is such a long
> way to go until I could be satisfied with the results, the course has created
> so much interest to continue in this direction.

Changes within the work setting

One thing that appears to surprise people is how they can apply the same ideas
and skills at many levels of their work. In some cases, they report that the greatest benefits are in the area of partnerships or teams as much as with patients:

> I have gone through phases of acquiring new skills (family trees, family
> legends, etc.) to looking at the whole consultation and work environment
> through a social constructionist lens.

> It has helped in the management of some very difficult staff members.

> I am much more keen on listening to other members of the team in particu-
> lar situations, and experienced it as a relief to be able to share my ideas.

It has made me think about how the team interacts internally and externally. It helps me to be able to understand other people's points of views. The influences on us are many and just being able to understand this is helpful.

I have really thought about my partnership and the way it works ... . It has crystallised my thoughts about my practice and how I will continue in the partnership and my role.

Here too, there can be problems. One of the most frequent difficulties that people report is that the course imposes an extra burden on their colleagues:

My partners are concerned that I am always 'rushing off' – and it's difficult to finish on time in order to get here.

They would rather I had been doing a surgery at the practice but are trying to be seen as tolerant of my quirky interest.

My partner has been supportive but apprehensive that I have had to change my work pattern to do the course.

My partners are unenthusiastically indulgent. They are aware of its importance to me – but not in what ways I think it will affect me.

My attendance here is guilt inducing! (Especially by the senior partner who feels left to carry the can.) Missing partners' meetings is a big problem. They would like to see positive benefits for patients and themselves.

My practice will be glad to see me back in surgery on Thursday afternoons. Relationships in the practice team, particularly with my partner, have improved, but I am unsure how much the rest of the team resented time for me attending the course.

Discussion

Primary care professionals greatly appreciate being in peer support groups, especially multidisciplinary ones. They appreciate the opportunity for 'all round' development: skills and ideas that they can apply across the whole range of their work. Such development deals with capability rather than competence, in other words with the ability for sustained and continuing change (Fraser and Greenhalgh 2000). Contrary to what one might expect, primary care professionals do not shrink from academic learning. Instead, they feel challenged and stimulated by it, and readily make the connections between abstract ideas and the complex realities of their everyday work.

Set against this, people who embark on this kind of learning face serious obstacles. Work pressure on themselves and their colleagues can set up serious tension. The kind of learning needed for significant technical and attitudinal change does not come quickly. Even the relative luxury of a half-day course over one to three terms may only be enough to whet their appetites and give them a sense of how much more could be achieved with more time.

Taken overall, the responses may suggest that a change is needed in the culture of primary care. It is a change towards recognising that professionals value education that brings about a fundamental reorientation in their approach to their work, and equips them with the skills to apply this. Primary care may need to be structured in future so that such learning can be offered more widely, and at greater length.

References

Fraser S and Greenhalgh T (2001) Complexity science: coping with complexity: educating for capability. *BMJ.* **323**: 799–803.

Hutchinson L (1999) Evaluating and researching the effectiveness of educational interventions. *BMJ.* **318**: 1267–9.

Kirkpatrick DI (1967) Evaluation of training. In: R Craig and I Bittel (eds) *Training and development handbook.* McGraw-Hill, New York.

Kiuttu J, Larivaara P, Väisänen E, Keinänen-Kiukaanniemi S and Oja H (1996) The effects of family systems medicine training on the practice orientations of general practitioners. *Fam Sys Health.* **14**: 453–62.

PART THREE

Theory

CHAPTER 14

From a patient-centred approach to a story-centred one

'All we can do is work with the vocabulary we have, while keeping our ears open for hints about how it might be expanded or revised.'
Richard Rorty (1989)

This section looks at different ways of understanding primary care. Its purpose is to highlight what is new and distinctive about a narrative approach from a theoretical point of view. More important, it proposes the case for moving towards a 'story-centred' approach as the main way of conceptualising what goes on in primary care in the early 21st century.

Such a proposal may seem audacious. It may also seem to undervalue or disqualify previous approaches. That is not the intention. As this chapter will make clear, a narrative approach, by its nature, sees all forms of understanding, and all stories, as evolutionary. Hence, no approach to primary care (including a narrative one) can be seen as ultimately authoritative. Any will contain insights fitted to their time and place. The case for moving towards a narrative-based approach is not that it is the only 'right' approach, but that it may be the right one for now. That theme runs throughout this section.

This chapter begins with a theoretical review of some of the primary care literature. In effect, that means the general practice consultation, since there is very little theoretical literature related to other primary care disciplines or to how teams or partnerships work. The review here focuses on a few central ideas that dominate general practice. This is followed by an account of how discomfort with these ideas keeps bubbling up within the profession. The remaining part of the chapter offers some examples of theoretical contributions from a narrative-based perspective. Taken altogether, the review is intended as a critique of conventional approaches and as a set of pointers towards a narrative approach to the consultation.

Chapter 15 looks at the Balint tradition, and the final chapter is entitled 'Towards a narrative-based model for primary care'. It can be read in its own right at any stage.

The consultation literature and its assumptions

There is a wide range of existing literature on the general practice consultation. In Britain, it includes some classic sociological studies such as those by Byrne and Long in the 1970s (Byrne and Long 1976) and by Tuckett and his team in the 1980s (Tuckett *et al.* 1985). Each of these used large-scale consultation research as a starting point for constructing models of how the general practice consultation ought to be conducted. In addition, there have been other models based either on literature reviews or personal experience or both. The most influential of these have probably been those by Pendleton (Pendleton *et al.* 1984) and Neighbour (1987).

Nationally and internationally, the total number of research articles and papers on the consultation is now vast. It comes from practitioners and from social scientists, and in some cases from both working together. A large number of studies are concerned with devising categories for consulting behaviour and testing GPs against these categories. In summary, and as Pendleton noted as long ago as 1984, there is a bewildering variety of models, and often the research does not lead to advice that is practical.

In spite of the multiplicity of approaches, certain typical beliefs appear to characterise virtually all the literature on the GP consultation. These beliefs are as follows.

- Patients arrive at their consultations with a fixed agenda (sometimes 'hidden'), which it is the doctor's task to discover.
- Their agendas can be determined by research interviews before or after the consultation.
- Each patient's preferences (for involvement in decision making, for example) are also fixed and the doctor needs to uncover them.
- The content of the consultation deserves more attention that the context. This means that issues such as time constraints or social rules are treated as incidentals rather than fundamental determinants of the consultation.

All these beliefs can be described as modernist or 'positivist'. They represent the idea that the consultation can be examined in much the same way that the physical sciences examine natural phenomena. In other words, there is a reality 'out there' in the consultation, and the diligent practitioner can be equipped to discern it, just as he or she learned to dissect a cadaver intelligently at medical school. By discovering this reality, the practitioner can work more effectively.

The discussion that follows shows how these beliefs operate in current approaches to the consultation. Necessarily, the examples from the consultation literature are selective, but in terms of their approach they are representative. The whole field is usefully summarised by Usherwood in his survey *Understanding the Consultation* (Usherwood 1999).

Assumption 1. Consultations should be patient centred

In an influential paper in the journal *Family Practice* in 1986, a team led by JH Levenstein described the 'patient-centred clinical method' (Levenstein *et al.* 1986). It set out a way of thinking and writing about the consultation that probably defines modern, humane, general practice:

> Every patient who seeks help has some expectations of the visit, not necessarily made explicit ... Every patient has some feelings about his problem or problems ... Although fear is an aspect of feeling, it is such a universal component of illness that we feel justified in giving it a separate heading ... Understanding the patient's expectations, feelings and fears will be specific for each patient ... Entry into the patient's world is a difficult art ... It also requires a skill in the practice of certain techniques ... The key to the patient-centred method, as its name implies, is to allow as much as possible to flow from the patient.

In terms of the task it addresses, the patient-centred approach is unimpeachable. Coming at a historical moment when patients' voices were first being heard on the social and political scene, it offered a corrective to paternalistic or authoritarian styles of consulting – and also to frankly inadequate ones where the physician responded to a problem that was quite different to the one the patient had actually brought. As a style of working, the patient-centred approach produces 'more humanistic interactions because patients are heard and understood in a different way' (Smith and Hoppe 1991).

Yet embedded within it are a number of unexamined assumptions that are now open to question. The first of these assumptions, as the sociologist David Armstrong has pointed out, is that the doctor has an unchallenged right to extend his or her 'gaze' into the area of the patient's own subjectivity (Armstrong 1982, 1984). Such approaches have become normative as 'good general practice', but in Armstrong's view this only confirms how well the medical profession has managed to extend its domain of inquiry and control. Even if one rejects such a severe view as this, it is clear that the patient-centred method carries some risk of intrusiveness. This may no longer be acceptable in a world where trust in doctors can no longer be assumed, and where the doctor's authority to make choices about which avenue of enquiry to pursue is open to challenge.

Another assumption that lies within the patient-centred approach is that the doctor should use a relatively passive technique that 'will allow as much as possible to flow from the patient'. This tenet of belief is no doubt influenced by a number of modern mental health approaches, including the use of silence in psychoanalysis and the empathic methods used by client-centred counsellors (Rogers 1951). What is missing, however, is a discussion of how to determine whether patients welcome this or whether they are experiencing it as withdrawal of involvement on the part of the doctor. One question to ask here is how the patient and practitioner might negotiate a satisfactory balance in the consultation – a balance that pays attention both to the patient's need for self-expression and to the doctor's professional responsibility. Another question is how doctors might judge how to modulate their consulting style from moment to moment in response to the specific events of each individual consultation.

From a narrative point of view, the most striking aspect of the patient-centred approach is that the patient's agenda is usually described as if it is something fixed and predetermined (Butler *et al.* 1992). Even if the agenda is described as 'hidden', there is always the implication that one can excavate for it and then hold it up to the light. In a book aptly entitled *Meetings with Experts*, Tuckett and his group express this belief with clarity:

> The patient's explanation of his problem (and to some extent his reasoning behind it) must be verbalised and elaborated together with his ideas and reasoning about what should be done and what consequences there may be. This will involve piecing together, elaborating and conceptualising the hints about their ideas that patients will drop. (Tuckett *et al.* 1985: 218)

In his survey of the consultation literature in general practice, Usherwood takes a similar view, incorporating a popular idea from medical anthropology about the importance of 'explanatory models' (Kleinman 1988):

> Without an understanding of the patient's health beliefs, the doctor will be in no position to provide an explanation that builds on the patient's existing explanatory model. At best the doctor will waste time by going over matters that the patient already knows; at worst she will fail to address potentially dangerous notions. (Usherwood 1999: 16)

In 20th-century terms, the views were highly enlightened ones. They emphasised how practitioners must enter the conceptual world of the patient before any effective conversation can be possible. Yet at the same time they may now be outdated in assuming that the doctor has the right to 'discover' the sole truth of any presentation (Kirmayer 1994). They are also restrictive. Many consultations defy a reductive interpretation in terms of 'uncovering the patient's agenda'. For example, how should one understand the hesitancies, uncertainties, discontinuities and confusion that characterise the stories that many patients bring? What is one to make of consultations where patients spontaneously recall extra symptoms, problems or thoughts that it was not their original intention to raise? From a narrative point of view, one way of answering these questions is by saying that patients are often not so much *bringing* an agenda as *seeking* one.

Assumption 2. Research can provide guidance on becoming patient centred

If the patient's agenda is seen as something predetermined and fixed, it is not surprising that researchers have generally assumed that they could establish beforehand exactly what patients wished to convey in any consultation, or could enquire afterwards whether they had managed to do so. Tuckett's team, for example, interviewed 328 patients and discovered this:

> The device of comparing what patients mentioned to doctors in their consultations with what they mentioned at interview, revealed that most of the patients studied did select what to tell their doctors. (Tuckett *et al.* 1985: 91)

They analysed the information that patients 'withheld', and found it to include symptoms, medication, depression and anxiety, and social troubles.

The power of research to elicit the agendas of patients and thus to highlight the inadequacies of doctors, has been a recurrent theme. Recently, a team led by Christine Barry from Brunel University, investigated 'patients' unvoiced agendas' and reached a conclusion very similar to Tuckett's:

> Patients have many needs, and when these are not voiced they cannot be addressed. Some of the poor outcomes in the case studies were related to unvoiced agenda items. This suggests that when patients and their needs are more fully articulated [sic] in the consultation better health care may be effected. (Barry *et al.* 2000)

Positivist studies like this do have a great deal to offer doctors. They sensitise them to areas of inattention, ignorance or discrimination. They point them towards the need to become better communicators in order to become more effective healers. Bochner encapsulates such findings with this perceptive remark:

> Communication difficulties in medical settings bear a remarkable resemblance to communication difficulties in cross-cultural settings . . . . Effectiveness depends on doctors becoming more sensitive to the frames of reference, linguistic usage, and life styles of the patients. (Bochner 1984)

At the same time, from a narrative point of view there is an obvious problem in using research interviews as a guide to consultations. The context of a consultation is not the same as the context of an interview. A consultation is shorter. It contains stresses for the doctor and patient that are not present when carrying out academic research. The story elicited in each situation is therefore likely to be completely different. The complexities of establishing what patients 'really' want from consultations, and the impossibility of ascertaining this with complete objectivity, can be demonstrated by asking a simple question: what might one discover if one did *research into the research*, asking patients whether there was anything they wanted to say to the researchers but withheld because of the way the researchers framed the questions, or because of time constraints, or for any other reason.

What may be needed instead of this positivist approach is a research methodology that looks at the linguistic process of consultations themselves. Such a methodology would need to explore how doctors can intervene at each particular juncture in a consultation, and whether or not this leads to a useful advance in the patient's story. In an exciting suggestion, Howard Brody argues that it should be possible to refine a narrative approach according to quite medical conventional measures of improvement:

> The available research suggests that such an approach can be extremely effective in relieving symptoms and ameliorating the effects of disease. The model can be further tested in a rigorous fashion and the results of that research used to refine the techniques of the physician–patient encounter and the joint construction of narrative. (Brody 1994)

These comments may point us towards a fascinating possibility: a convergence of narrative practice with outcome research that is acceptable within the medical community. It may be possible to use conventional tools such as the Consultation Satisfaction Questionnaire or Patient Enablement Instrument to test whether the right stories are being facilitated (Stevenson 1993, Howie *et al.* 2000)

Assumption 3. Patients have preferences

In recent years, a favourite question for researchers into general practice has been: 'What kind of doctors do patients want?' (Little *et al.* 2001). There has been much curiosity about whether individual patients prefer their doctors to be authoritative in their pronouncements or to take a more enabling stance. There is, for example, a classic study by Thomas showing that patients preferred definite diagnoses to vague ones (Thomas 1987), work by Savage and Armstrong in 1990 showing that more patients preferred authoritative doctors (Savage and Armstrong 1990) and research by McKinstry ten years later demonstrating that patients vary in their desire to be involved in decision making, according to class, age, education, usual doctor's style and smoking (McKinstry 2000). Yet once again researchers have seen patients' preferences (and indeed doctors' consulting behaviour) as something static and unvarying, available for discovery but not influence. Middleton and McKinley express this view by proposing an elaborate schema based on undiluted positivism:

> Each patient's preference for partnership in the consultation is located within a multi-dimensional framework, the axes of which embrace differing desires and needs for information, assistance with its interpretation, and involvement in the final decision making. The patient's preference for sharing or being directed must be determined on each axis. (Middleton and McKinley 2000)

Once again, this kind of analysis is based on the modernist idea that there is a single absolute truth in each situation that is waiting to be discovered. This is now at odds with a more contemporary view that any encounter involves two particular individuals who each bring their own contexts and subjective preferences to bear on it, and will therefore create a conversation that is entirely unique. What is also missing from such an analysis is the idea that the doctor–patient conversation might itself be a means of inviting patients to reconsider at each moment the position they might wish to take on any of these axes. If this is so, we now need to discover how to explore flexibility in consultations, so that we neither ignore patients' preferences nor assume that these are always rigid.

Assumption 4. Content is more important than context

Every working GP who studies the consultation literature must notice the absence of almost any reference to time constraints. Similarly, social scientists must be puzzled by the way that writers set standards for consultations, without reference to the social, political or moral values from which these are derived. Anyone approaching the literature from a narrative point of view will also become aware of the number of 'ex cathedra' statements telling doctors how to structure the content of their consultations. For example, Tuckett's team determined at the start of their study that a doctor should offer the following information in *every* consultation (Tuckett *et al.* 1985):

- the 'diagnostic significance' of a problem
- the appropriate treatment action to deal with a problem
- the appropriate preventive measures that may be necessary to forestall or lessen future episodes
- the implications or wider social and emotional consequences of problems and their treatment.

Kurtz and Silverman propose a structure for each consultation as follows (Kurtz and Silverman 1996):

1 Initiating the session.
2 Gathering information.
3 Examination.
4 Explanation and planning.
5 Closing the session.

Neighbour also offers a similar check list of what should be done in every consultation (Neighbour 1987). So do Stott and Davis (1979). Usherwood asserts:

> It is a good discipline to try to address an issue of health promotion at least once during every consultation. Examples include reviewing current immunisation status, performing a cervical smear, checking the blood pressure or enquiring about smoking and alcohol consumption. (Usherwood 1999: 18).

He makes no reference to any need to harmonise this activity with the rest of the encounter with the patient, and he seems unaware of the many critiques that have been launched against 'surveillance medicine' generally (Davies 1984, Williams and Boulton 1988, Sachs 1995, Armstrong 1995).

Once again, there is clearly merit in all these proposals. Many of them contain extremely valuable guidance on how to facilitate patients' self-expression, or how to modulate advice or explanations in response to feedback. At the same time, there is a selective focus in them. For example, they all offer advice to practitioners about how to conduct the consultation, without any reference to external factors such as the pressure of work, the resources of the practice, the relationships between team members or the constraints of money and clinical targets. There is also a certain unexamined paternalism in these kinds of guidance. In particular, they all take it for granted that the doctor should hold on to the sole authority for the overall shape, division and progress of consultations, rather than allowing these to be sculpted jointly with the patient. What they do not acknowledge is that patients may want as much control over the process of the encounter as the content. They may want to be heard rather than herded.

The sociologist PM Strong has discussed the way that 'communication skills' are taught to doctors and nurses. In a compelling critique, he has noted how such 'skills' inevitably contain their own external rules and logic, yet at the same time these are never highlighted or discussed. In effect, the true rules of 'good' consulting are rendered invisible and hence unchallengeable. He makes this point:

> ...[The] communications approach, by emphasising the individual, renders the organisation transparent; its actual workings, organisational procedures and resources, the social settings and roles of the participants, all of these are simply assumed. At the same time ... organisational purposes are still present but in covert and thus uninspected form .... Thus 'communication' is used in a very special sense. It does not refer at all to the myriad ways in which doctor and patient both present their behaviour and read that of the other, as each attempt to make sense of and to control the situation ... (Strong 1979: 5)

In contrast to the communications approach, the narrative approach offers a view of the consultation as an event that is entirely determined by its contexts. It openly acknowledges the limits that these contexts impose. It suggests that this acknowledgement can be shared transparently with the patient. It also suggests that patients should be allowed to exert their own influence over what happens, so that the consultation becomes an act of co-creation rather than compulsion. Rather than following guidelines, narrative practitioners alter their behaviour according to what is going on from moment to moment in the conversation.

Epistemological discomfort in the general practice literature

While there are many voices in general practice asserting the primacy of 'the patient's agenda' and of the 'patient-centred method', there have always been voices expressing discomfort at this linear way of conceptualising doctor–patient conversations.

Sometimes, the same people put forward both viewpoints at different times. For example, Byrne and Long, the pioneers of large-scale GP consultation research, take a prescriptive approach in their work, with long check lists of desirable interviewing behaviour and a complex points system. Yet in passing they also propose an important distinction between a conventional medical style of interviewing and a counselling style where questions are regarded as *effects* of the previous information as well as *causes* of the information still to come (Byrne and Long 1976).

The same struggle – between codifying the consultation process and a more fluid way of viewing it – is evident in the work of David Pendleton. In the context of his literature review, he writes in fairly conventional terms:

> . . . satisfaction of the patient is more likely when the doctor discovers and deals with the patient's concerns and expectations; when the doctor's manner communicates warmth, interest and concern about the patient; when the doctor volunteers a lot of information and explains things to the patient in terms that are understood.

However, his conclusion is unmistakably an interactional one:

> A formulation of consultation processes in terms of social interaction would clarify the role of the consultation as a transaction or mutual social influence process and would lead to an expectation that the consultation would bring about changes in their participants. (Pendleton 1984: 46)

A similar approach is taken by two other authors, Paul Freeling and Conrad Harris. Their model is based mainly on Eric Berne's system of transactional analysis, although they also refer to Salvador Minuchin's structural assessment of families. Their conclusion reaches ideas that echo Pendleton's:

> . . . in medicine no consultation with a conscious patient can ever be merely diagnostic: it always has some effects on the patient's subsequent feelings and behaviour. (Freeling and Harris 1984: 130)

Similarly, as we have seen, Usherwood takes a fairly prescriptive approach to the consultation but he also quotes Little's critique of such an approach:

> When clinicians 'take' a medical history they turn the patient's narrative to text, removing the discourse from the patient's lived experience. Doctors assume a set of editorial functions, determined by their need to observe linguistic conventions that may be entirely alien to the patient. (Little 1995)

Usherwood himself then goes further:

> Doctors do more than this. Through their questions and other utterances, they coax the patient to produce the kind of narrative they want ... . Indeed, the very story that the patient produces will reflect in part the doctor's interpretation and consequent responses. The danger is not that the doctor influences the patient's narrative – that is unavoidable – but that he does so without understanding. Doctors need to reflect continually on their values and prejudices, and to be aware of how these impact directly on their clinical encounters. (Usherwood 1999: 66)

Comments like these occur throughout the literature. They often leave the impression that researchers have emerged with a sense of discomfort about existing epistemological paradigms for understanding the consultation.

Perhaps the most audacious, and poetic, analysis of the problem and its potential solution comes from Marshall Marinker:

> What if the encounter itself came to be seen ... not as a process but as an outcome? If the consultation then can be at one and the same time a process in the sense that it is concerned with diagnosis and management of a clinical problem, and an outcome in that it represents an end in itself, the definitive answer to the question that it poses, we will require new forms of analysis and new criteria for judgement. Such a quantum leap in thinking is unlikely to be achieved in the cosy confines of, say, general practice or social psychology. But it may come from the confusion and perhaps even the fusion of both. That may be the distant prize for patient care which we start to win now when we teach about the consultation, when we puzzle over the communication, and when we have tried to measure its dimensions and to interpret what it is that we are about. This could form the basis of a subversive/gnostic approach to the consultation which hums through the literature but is never sung aloud. (Marinker 1985)

Narrative ideas from family therapy: an alternative set of assumptions

As the Introduction made clear, the narrative ideas that underlie this book are mostly taken from contemporary thinking in family therapy. In its turn, that thinking has been deeply influenced by ideas about narrative from the social sciences and the humanities.

In contrast with some of the ideas that organise so much work on the GP consultation, different assumptions now prevail in the world of family therapy. Family therapists see their consultations as interactive and evolutionary. Unlike most people currently working in primary care, they regard patients' problems not as the *end point* for a process of detection but as the *starting point* for a creative conversation leading to a new narrative. Most family therapists now work according to a narrative-based set of assumptions. These include the following.

- Language does not describe reality, it creates it.
- Problems are open to multiple stories.
- Some stories are better than others.
- You cannot achieve objectivity but you can expand your awareness of subjectivity.

The rest of this chapter examines these assumptions in turn. It illustrates them with quotations from eminent family therapists. It draws attention to the contrast with the assumptions that govern patient-centred medicine, and therefore suggests an alternative way of approaching the primary care consultation.

Assumption 1. Language not only describes reality, it also creates it

According to many contemporary therapists, patients' problems do not have an objective existence. Essentially, they are the results of previous conversations, and they will exist only for as long as other conversations continue to define them as problems. This kind of view is characteristic of the movement known as *social constructionism* (*see* Introduction). The following quotation from the leading family therapist Lynn Hoffman, although rather dense in its prose, puts the point forcefully:

> Social constructionism posits an evolving set of meanings that emerge unendingly from the interactions between people. These meanings are not skull-bound and may not exist inside what we think of as an individual 'mind'. They are part of a general flow of constantly changing narratives .... The development of concepts is a fluid process, socially derived. I think it is particularly helpful for the therapist to think of problems as stories that people have agreed to tell themselves. (Hoffman 1990)

To call a problem 'a story' is not to minimise or dismiss it. Quite the contrary: this way of looking at problems points toward a way of helping with them. Social constructionism invites us to notice the social processes by which 'problems' become labelled as such – processes in which we ourselves play a part as practitioners. It cautions us against pathologising people, even when they invite us to do so. It might prompt practitioners in primary care to regard problems as less concrete, and more open to dissolution and reconstruction, than we might otherwise have realised.

Assumption 2. Problems are open to multiple stories

Because family therapists see problems in terms of the stories told about them, they also argue that every problem is open to many different descriptions or stories. They do not reject familiar ways of looking at the world – ideas like problems and agendas, diagnoses and explanations. However, they regard all of these as provisional descriptions only. They also regard all narratives and all definitions as open to exploration and challenge. Indeed, they see this as the task of all therapy.

Carlos Sluzki (1992) suggests that the key idea governing therapeutic explorations should be the attempt to transform narratives by asking questions that offer the possibility of shifts in a number of dimensions, including the following:

- shifts between a static definition of events, symptoms, traits or people, and active descriptions of exactly who does what
- shifts between a story devoid of historical roots and context and one with a starting point, scenario and evolution
- shifts between a story centred in the assumed cause or origin and one that includes its ongoing effects
- shifts between attribution of intent to someone and a discussion of the effect of their behaviour
- shifts between attributions of craziness, unreasonableness, incompetence and illogicality to people and attributions that assume saneness, reasonableness, competence and logic
- shifts between assumptions about hidden meanings of events and accounts of those events.

One way of looking at Sluzki's list of suggestions is as a guide for 'story-weaving'. The practitioner takes the patient's initial description, which may be a very negative or repetitive one, and exercises a kind of systematic curiosity about its unexplained or unexplored aspects. The process of doing so helps to transform one story into another, and hence one view of reality into another.

One illustration of how this might be done in primary care appears in an extraordinary case description by Tomm and Lannaman (1988). They give an account of how Karl Tomm helped a couple where the husband was initially attached to the idea that his depression had an organic cause, while his wife was more willing to entertain the possibility that it had a connection with family events and circumstances. The therapist remained neutral concerning his own beliefs (or lack of them) with respect to the 'causes' of depression. Through a process of sympathetic questioning, both husband and wife became more flexible in the range of descriptions they were willing to offer concerning what 'the problem' was, and how it had come about. This had a marked and sustained effect in relieving the man's depression.

Assumption 3. Some stories are better than others

A naive reading of a narrative-based approach might suggest that, since problems are entirely negotiable, any new story is fine and all new stories are equal. In fact, there is a strong emphasis in family therapy on the aesthetic and practical value of the story *to the patient.* It is the patient who must judge if the story 'fits' and offers a useful way forward. Amundson suggests that a therapist should be prepared to use a variety of theoretical models for generating new ideas, new questions and new stories, and should judge their value not by their apparent internal coherence but by their pragmatic consequences in each case (Amundson 1996).

The emphasis on producing better stories for patients also leads to a highly developed attentiveness to language. If, as is argued, new realities are created by language itself, the onus is clearly on the clinician to give the minutest concentration to the words the patient uses, and to their smallest nuances. Without understanding the precise import of the patient's descriptions, there is no possibility of opening up new ones. As a result, there is an emphasis on noticing the exact feedback to the therapist's questions. This leads many therapists to anatomise the utterances of consultations (often using video afterwards) to a degree that makes general practice consulting seem a very raw art indeed.

An excellent example of this discipline appears in an article by Reimers. He offers a precise verbal analysis of various examples of 'talking at cross purposes' in family therapy. He suggests that such moments can offer very valuable indications of how exactly the patients wish to be understood. In a striking conclusion, he suggests that an absence of misunderstanding in consultations 'may even be a warning that clients have themselves adjusted or even resigned themselves too well to a therapy which is not serving them properly' (Reimers 1999).

Many people in primary care might recognise this as an apt description of certain long-term relationships with patients that have become politely stale or imperceptibly inert.

Assumption 4. You cannot achieve objectivity but you can expand your awareness of subjectivity

At the core of a narrative approach is the notion of 'intersubjectivity'. This term encompasses the idea that no one is capable of defining the nature of the other person's experience. Instead, all that is ever possible is the engagement of two subjective stories, each formed by the individual circumstances of personal history, family background, gender, ethnicity, culture, profession and so forth. Thus, no one is ever in a position to say authoritatively: '*You are suffering from X.*' All they are capable of saying, in effect, is: '*My own personal prejudices lead me to describe your condition by using the word X.*' This idea has now gained a central status not only within family therapy but in the humanities, and within large areas of the social sciences too (Guba and Lincoln 1994). In a therapeutic context, the idea can be summed up as follows:

> Therapy occurs when the prejudices of the family and the therapist interact. The kind of relationship that will emerge also derives from the encounter of the prejudices of the family and therapist. So, from our systemic perspective, it is not the content of the prejudice, but the relationship between the prejudices of the client and therapist that is the heart of the therapy. (Cecchin *et al.* 1994)

At first sight, this might seem a fatalistic position to take. It might even appear to disqualify practitioners from practising therapy, medicine or indeed any other activity that purports to offer help. In the view of social constructionists, however, an understanding of intersubjectivity is a necessary step on the path to honesty in the consultation, ethical professional behaviour and power sharing with the patient. It enables people to take responsibility for their own individual actions and choices.

Intersubjectivity has its counterpart in *reflexivity*: an ability to reflect on, articulate and share the subjective nature of what is going on. Reflexivity demands a process of self-interrogation regarding the beliefs and assumptions leading to a particular line of questioning in the consultation. Reflexivity involves a willingness to 'bring the context into the room', as described in Chapter 2. For instance, a practitioner might ask questions about the other person's reality and how it was different: '*I'm a white male professional and you're a black female immigrant. How do you think that affects the way we might each see your problem?*'

Reflexivity may also involve being 'up front' about one's own beliefs, particularly where these are at odds with the patient's. An example of this would be to say: '*As someone who sees children a great deal, I believe that most of them are hurt by their parents separating, but I'm interested that you don't see things this way.*'

From 'the patient's view' to 'the creation of new narrative': the next step forward?

Armstrong has argued that medicine has gone through a series of transformations in the past three centuries: from an enlightenment discourse that described lesions in the body, to a modernist one which spoke of lesions in the mind, to a critical one that now places an emphasis on 'the patient's view' (Armstrong 1984). In some places, such as parts of the hospital service, the critical view is still making its advances against the steadfast resistance of many practitioners. Yet within primary care, the emphasis on 'the patient's view' seems to have become an accepted orthodoxy.

As this chapter has shown by its analysis of two different sets of assumptions, a narrative approach challenges the current orthodoxy of primary care in its turn. It invites practitioners to transform their view of their encounters with patients, from an observational one involving the search for objectivity, to one involving the interaction of two subjective stories, each determined by its own contexts. In terms of a theory, the narrative approach offers an important way forward in a number of respects. It places practitioners and patients on a more level footing, in a way that is more consistent with a contemporary understanding of patients' rights and professionals' duties. It offers an identical theoretical framework for understanding both the patient's reality and the professional's, rather than assuming that each should be understood in terms decided by the latter. It provides a single coherent view of all the different kinds of encounters with patients, by all its various kinds of practitioners. It also suggests a unitary way of conceptualising the whole range of both clinical and non-clinical activity in primary care.

Inevitably, it also gives rise to some important questions. How can one introduce an approach that is inherently subtle and subversive into a professional world that is mainly concrete in its thinking and is closely connected with social forms of control? How far should one go in pushing the more 'postmodern' versions of narrative thinking, including those that suggest that phenomena like strokes and death should be considered as mere consensual 'stories'? How might one integrate a view of the world as composed from stories, with a scientific approach to knowledge and expertise? These are crucial theoretical challenges for a narrative approach, and they need to be addressed. The final chapter addresses these questions, particularly the last one. Before that discussion, however, there is another view of primary care that has to be considered: the view of the Balint tradition. That is the subject of the next chapter.

References

Amundson J (1996) Why pragmatics are probably enough for now. *Fam Proc.* **35**: 473–86.

Armstrong D (1982) The doctor–patient relationship, 1930–80. In: P Wright and A Treacher (eds) *The Problem of Medical Knowledge*. Edinburgh University Press, Edinburgh.

Armstrong D (1984) The patient's view. *Soc Sci Med.* **18**: 737–44.

Armstrong D (1995) The rise of surveillance medicine. *Soc Health Illn.* **17**: 393–404.

Barry CA, Bradley CP, Britten N, Stevenson FA and Barber N (2000) Patients' unvoiced agendas in general practice consultations: qualitative study. *BMJ.* **320**: 1246–50.

Bochner S (1984) Doctors, patients and their cultures. In: D Pendleton and J Hasler (eds) *Doctor Patient Communication*. Academic Press, London.

Brody H (1994) 'My story is broken; can you help me fix it?' Medical ethics and the joint construction of narrative. *Lit Med.* **13**: 79–92.

Butler NM, Campion PD and Cox AD (1992) Exploration of doctor and patient agendas in general practice consultations. *Soc Sci Med.* **35**: 1145–55.

Byrne PS and Long BEL (1976) *Doctors Talking to Patients*. Her Majesty's Stationery Office, London.

Cecchin G, Lane G and Ray W (1994) *The Cybernetics of Prejudices in the Practice of Psychotherapy*. Karnac, London.

Davies C (1984) General practitioners and the pull of prevention. *Soc Health Illn.* **6**: 267–89.

Freeling P and Harris CM (1984) *The Doctor Patient Relationship*. Longman, London.

Guba E and Lincoln Y (1994) Competing paradigms in qualitative research. In: NK Denzin and Y Lincoln (eds) *Handbook of Qualitative Research*. Sage, London.

Hoffman L (1990) Constructing realities: an art of lenses. *Fam Proc.* **29**: 1–12.

Howie JGR, Heaney DJ, Maxwell M and Walker JJ (2000) Developing a 'consultation quality index' (CQI) for use in general practice. *Fam Pract.* **17**: 455–61.

Kirmayer L (1994) Improvisation and authority in illness meaning. *Cult Med Psychiatry.* **18**: 183–214.

Kleinman A (1988) *The Illness Narratives: suffering, healing and the human condition*. Basic Books, New York.

Kurtz S and Silverman J (1996) The Calgary–Cambridge Observation Guides: an aid to defining the curriculum and organizing the teaching in communication training programmes. *Med Educ.* **30**: 83–9.

Levenstein JH, McCracken EC, McWhinney IR, Stewart MA and Brown JB (1986) The patient-centred clinical method. 1. A model for the doctor-patient interaction in family medicine. *Fam Pract.* **3**: 24–30.

Little M (1995) *Humane Medicine.* Cambridge University Press, Cambridge.

Little P, Everitt H, Williamson I *et al.* (2001) Preferences of patients for patient centred approach to consultation in primary care: observational study. *BMJ.* **322**: 468–72.

Marinker M (1985) Communication in general practice: new consultations for old. In: D Pendleton and J Hasler (eds) *Doctor Patient Communication.* Academic Press, London.

McKinstry B (2000) Do patients wish to be involved in decision making in the consultation? A cross-sectional survey with video vignettes. *BMJ.* **321**: 867–71.

Middleton JF and McKinley RD (2000) What kind of partnership in the consultation? *BMJ.* **321**: 268–9.

Neighbour R (1987) *The Inner Consultation.* MTP Press, Lancaster.

Pendleton D (1984) Doctor–patient communication: a review. In: D Pendleton and J Hasler (eds) *Doctor Patient Communication.* Academic Press, London.

Pendleton D, Schofield T, Tate P and Havelock P (1984) *The Consultation: an approach to learning and teaching.* Oxford University Press, Oxford.

Reimers S (1999) 'Good morning, Sir!' 'Axe handle': talking at cross purposes in family therapy. *J Fam Ther.* **21**: 360–76.

Rogers P (1951) *Client-centred Therapy.* Houghton Mifflin, Boston.

Rorty R (1989) *Contingency, Irony and Solidarity.* Cambridge University Press, Cambridge.

Sachs L (1995) Is there a pathology of prevention? The implications of visualising the invisible in screening programmes. *Cult Med Psychiatry.* **19**: 503–25.

Savage R and Armstrong D (1990) Effect of a general practitioner's consulting style on patient's satisfaction: qualitative analysis. *BMJ.* **318**: 372–6.

Sluzki C (1992) Transformations, a blueprint for narrative changes in therapy. *Fam Proc.* **31**: 217–30.

Smith RC and Hoppe RB (1991) The patient's story: integrating the patient- and physician-centred approaches to interviewing. *Ann Intern Med.* **115**: 470–7.

Stevenson C (1993) Combining quantitative and qualitative methods in evaluating a course of family therapy. *J Fam Ther.* **15**: 205–24.

Stott N and Davis R (1979) The exceptional potential in each primary care consultation. *J Roy Coll Gen Pract.* **29**: 201–5.

Strong PM (1979) *The Ceremonial Order of the Clinic: parents, doctors and medical bureaucracies.* Routledge and Kegan Paul, London.

Thomas KB (1987) General practice consultations: is there any point in being positive? *BMJ*. **294**: 1200–2.

Tomm K and Lannaman J (1988) Questions as interventions. *Fam Ther Networker*. **12**: 38–41.

Tuckett D, Boulton M, Olson C and Williams A (1985) *Meetings Between Experts*. Tavistock, London.

Usherwood T (1999) *Understanding the Consultation: evidence, theory and practice*. Open University Press, Buckingham.

Williams A and Boulton M (1988) Thinking prevention: concepts and constructs in general practice. In: M Lock and D Gordon (eds) (1988) *Biomedicine Examined*. Kluwer, Dordrecht.

Balint and narrative:
a comparison

'There are many cases in which – though the signs of a confusion of tongues are painfully present – there is apparently no open controversy.'
Michael Balint (1957)

This chapter offers a comparison between a narrative-based approach and an approach influenced by Balint and the Balint tradition. It looks from a theoretical perspective at points of convergence and also at points of divergence between the two approaches. As with the previous chapter, the focus is not on an exhaustive review of the literature, but on a reasoned critique. The overall aim is to highlight the characteristics of a narrative-based approach. It is also to propose how a narrative approach might offer a way forward for primary care, going beyond what the Balint tradition has to offer without devaluing the contribution it has made.

Why consider Balint?

There are several reasons why it is worth making a specific comparison with Balint. First, there is a tendency to lump together any reflective approaches to the psychological or conceptual aspects of general practice under the rather lazy heading of 'Balint'. This confusion needs unscrambling. As mentioned in Chapter 10, some people inevitably assume that the approach we teach is connected to the Balint movement, as both originated at the Tavistock Clinic. In fact, the two have different histories, ideas and educational styles.

There is a far more important reason for making a comparison. Balint's work, and that of his followers, probably represents the only attempt that has ever been made to offer a single coherent theoretical framework to describe all the work that GPs do. The Balint tradition continues to dominate postgraduate training, or a significant section of it, in many countries. Although the number of formal Balint groups now active in Britain is small (Balint *et al.* 1993), many of the working conventions of these groups are deeply embedded in primary care training. These include free-ranging discussion of individual cases, with an emphasis on the psychological aspects of people's problems, and on the doctor–patient relationship. Any proposal for an alternative conceptual framework for thinking about primary care must stand comparison with Balint's, and must offer an intelligent critique of it.

Theoretical discussion of the Balint tradition has some particular limitations. One of these is that it can make 'the Balint approach' look entirely homogeneous, when this is clearly not the case. We cannot know how every Balint group, or every group leader, has behaved. There is no doubt that the Balint movement has evolved historically so that it is in some ways unrecognisably different from the recorded practice of its founder or his immediate followers (Clyne 1961). In addition, much activity that now takes place in the name of Balint, both in Britain and around the world, bears very little resemblance to what the leaders of the 'official' Balint movement would recognise as fitting that description (Balint *et al.* 1993). Nowadays, the movement is a very protean one, so that the meaning of 'the Balint approach' seems to depend very much on who you are and where you are (Sackin 2001). It may be necessary to spell out that this tradition, as it exists today, is not always synonymous either with the man or the movement. It may also be important to point out that many people who have had a brief exposure to some Balint training may not practise in the same way as the more highly trained group leaders.

Another problem in discussing 'the Balint approach' is that Balint and his followers have always explicitly avoided any specific technical advice about how to conduct consultations. Although many practitioners who have been influenced by the movement may have extrapolated similar conclusions from their case discussions with regard to how to consult with patients, it is impossible to point to any particular style of consulting behaviour and say for certain that it has the official imprimatur of Balint.

One response to these limitations might be to avoid any critique of 'the Balint approach' on the grounds that it is so nebulous. Yet there does seem to be a recognisable way of thinking about primary care, and of consulting in that setting, that one might fairly call Balintian. These elements can be traced both to the Balint movement and to the writings of Balint himself. These are the elements addressed in this chapter.

Nearly all the discussion here concerns the GP consultation, since that is the focus of the theoretical literature (although the Balint movement has now extended its work to other professions, including practice nurses and counsellors). However, the discussion may be applicable to other disciplines in primary care and to other aspects of primary care work.

Balint and narrative-based primary care: points of convergence

There are many points of theoretical convergence between Balint's ideas and a narrative-based approach. Many of these no doubt arise from the nature of the work in primary care itself.

Michael Balint took a particular interest in the potential of general practice as a therapeutic milieu. In his book *The Doctor, his Patient and the Illness*, he offered a detailed understanding of the work of general practice (Balint 1957). The approach taken is in many ways a narrative approach. Balint's book is full of stories about patients. So are most of the books and articles that have emerged from the Balint movement. The Balint movement takes stories seriously. It regards them not as mere 'anecdotes' but as the very stuff of general practice. There is an implicit recognition that doctors need to tell stories just as patients do, and that they especially need to do this when they have encounters that are unsettling or unresolved. Balint himself first instituted case discussion seminars for GPs – so called Balint groups – to meet that need (Gosling and Turquet 1964). These groups were the first systematic attempt to set up any kind of postgraduate learning or clinical supervision for primary care.

Balint saw the GP consultation as a form of therapy (Balint 1957: 9). He invited GPs to develop their capacity to listen and understand, 'using that understanding so that it should have a therapeutic effect'. He suggested doctors should try to 'predict with a fair amount of accuracy' what sort of effect any intervention might have. At the same time, he conceded that the effects of anything spoken or not spoken in the consultation could be unpredictable (Balint 1957: Ch 10). He was realistic about the limits of psychotherapy in the GP surgery, but his respect for GPs and their work setting enabled him to see that there were many things that a GP might do that would be inadvisable, impossible or unthinkable for a psychiatrist (Balint 1957: Ch 13). In the early years of the Balint movement, there was a fashion for a kind of limited psychotherapy in the surgery. GPs were encouraged to set aside protected time, perhaps outside normal opening hours, to deal with cases that were emotionally demanding (Salinsky 1993). In general, however, enthusiasm for this style of working has waned, and there has been much more of a focus on how to work reflectively in the very short moments of contact that GPs generally have for their patients (Balint and Norell 1973, Elder and Samuel 1987, Elder 1990).

One consistent theme is that the therapeutic relationship between patient and GP develops over time and through many successive short episodes of shared commitment – something that Balint nicely described as a 'mutual investment company'. Balint also placed an important emphasis on language in its wider sense. In particular, he identified the fact that doctors and patients often behave as if they are speaking about the same things when in fact they are not – a point highlighted by the epigraph to this chapter. He also cautioned against the tendency of doctors to try and convert patients to their own views of the world – a kind of medical evangelism that he entitled 'the apostolic function'.

In his theoretical writing, Balint paid attention to the wider context of GP work, especially the GP–consultant relationship. He perceptively identified the 'collusion of anonymity' whereby both GPs and hospital doctors avoid the emotional and moral ownership of the patients in their care (Balint 1957: Ch 7). He was a compelling commentator on the way that conventional medical thinking could constrain and distort GP work. He noted that the traditional form of 'direct questioning' taught in medical school actually militates against developing the doctor–patient relationship, so that 'structurising the doctor–patient relationship on the pattern of a physical examination inactivates the processes [that the GP] wants to observe as they can happen only in a two person collaboration' (Balint 1957: 121).

Interestingly, Balint was one of the first people to understand the need for basic research to take place into the nature of general practice and the conversations that took place there. He conceptualised the activity of his GP seminars primarily as research aimed at continually generating new understanding and new theory (Balint 1957: Ch 18). He realised that GPs, and the psychoanalysts who worked with them in their case seminars, would need to develop new kinds of description of the work, quite distinct from the conventional medical descriptions of cases. He believed that the research activity of his groups should be inseparable from a coherent and seamless infrastructure for general practice that would involve not only case discussion but also training, supervision, case consultancy and onward referral. This belief is clear from Balint's two successive prefaces to his book and from his own appendices. It is spelled out most clearly in the appendix by John Sutherland, then medical director of the Tavistock, entitled 'An additional role for the psychological clinic'. It is a depressing indictment of secondary mental healthcare in Britain that this central trend in Balint's thinking has so often been ignored.

Balint and narrative-based primary care: where they diverge

In spite of all these similarities, a narrative-based approach offers considerable difference from a Balintian approach. The following section addresses four interconnected areas where this appears to be the case. These are:

- questions
- emotions
- contexts
- interpretations.

Questions

Broadly speaking, Balint himself disapproved of asking too many questions in the consultation. One of his most often-quoted remarks is: 'If you ask questions, you will get answers, but hardly anything else' (Horder 2001). The same attitude is implicit or explicit throughout most of the writings of his followers (Sackin 1994). From accounts of Balint seminars, it appears that most group leaders actively discourage participants from asking too many questions of the case presenters in the groups themselves. They also discourage asking too many questions in consultations with patients. This guidance reflects the psychoanalytic approach, which places an emphasis on reflective comments and silence in preference to further enquiry. It is in marked contrast to the approach taken in a narrative-based approach, where questioning is regarded as a prerequisite for effective interviewing.

At one level, the difference in attitude towards questioning is a purely technical one. At another level, it points to a fundamental difference in theoretical approach. It represents the difference between a model based on observing psychic function and another based on promoting interactions. From a psychoanalytically oriented point of view, questions are an intrusion. They interrupt the patient's chain of associations and can impede emotional expression. From a narrative point of view, however, they are an essential therapeutic intervention. They are the principal means of helping patients to move from a linear to a more interactional understanding of their problem, and from a static to a dynamic one (Payne 2000) They are a way of changing old, repetitive stories into new ones.

Emotions

Another difference between the two approaches is in their attitudes to emotions. In the Balint tradition, there often appears to be an assumption that intimacy, close personal engagement and perhaps even emotional catharsis are desirable in encounters with patients. In Balint's own writings, there are several accounts of GPs encouraging patients to disclose details of their sexual habits and fantasies – including, in one case, fantasies about the doctor himself (Balint 1957: 203). The emphasis on sexuality and on disclosure has been greatly tempered in the Balint movement since then, in line with wider social awareness of the problems of such enquiries. However, there has always been a premium placed on close personal engagement with patients' experiences. A much quoted example is the so-called 'flash': 'an intense moment of mutual awareness in doctor and patient, resulting in the possibility of change or enrichment in the working relationship' (Gill 1979). Recent theoretical writing from the Balint movement also places a value on personal engagement, sometimes framing this in terms of doctors learning to lower their own emotional defences (Salinsky and Sackin 2001). Whatever the intention of such thinking might be in terms of behaviour in the consultation (and this is never exactly spelled out), it does appear to have an observable effect in the tendency of some practitioners to explore emotion 'for its own sake'. This is a habit we have observed perhaps more than any other in practitioners who report that they have been influenced directly or indirectly by the Balint tradition.

A narrative-based approach values intimacy and emotion. However, there are some crucial questions to be asked in this area. One question is whether strong emotion is ever valuable for its own sake. For example, when a doctor hands the patient a tissue to wipe away tears, it can be a very moving moment, but it begs the question: what have the tears achieved? Is it merely a transient release of emotion or is it a more substantial change? If not, could change have been achieved in another way – perhaps through an intervention promoting empowerment?

Another question about personal engagement and emotion concerns the risk of harming patients by being intrusive. There are many occasions when patients do need to disclose painful things, but there are also occasions when this is not the case. It may also be impossible to deal with powerful emotions adequately in the context of a general practice consultation – because the time is too short or the external pressures too great. In the view of many family therapists, practitioners who seek emotional intimacy may end up by reinforcing stories of helplessness rather than creating opportunities to change these. A more neutral interviewing style may be more effective, as well as safer, in allowing people to develop an alternative story over time.

There is an interesting comparison to be made here between a Balintian approach and patient-centred medicine. As Chapter 14 made clear, patient-centred medicine represents a considerable advance on authoritarian modes of consulting, but nowadays might be seen as too prescriptive in its view of how to elicit the patient's story and therefore liable to reinforce that story instead of developing it. In the same way, the Balint tradition has rightly insisted that the emotional dimension of people's experience should be brought into view, but it may fall short on examining how and why this should be done, or how the doctor should proceed when it does.

Contexts

People who follow Balint appear to pay most attention to one context: the doctor–patient relationship. Although there are passing references in the literature to other contexts, such as GP practices or the wider culture, these are always subordinated to a discussion of the doctor–patient relationship itself. This very precise focus can also be traced to the psychoanalytic theories that informed Balint's thinking, and especially to the concept of the unconscious mind being revealed through 'counter-transference'. (This refers to the idea that any feelings stirred up in the doctor can reveal underlying truths about the patient's real problem.)

This single-minded focus is most striking in the writing of Balint himself. To take one example, there is a lengthy discussion in *The Doctor, his Patient and the Illness* concerning a patient who is a refugee. In passing, we learn: 'She originally came from central Europe, where she lost her husband through Hitler.' In the remaining discussion, there is no further reference to this (Balint 1957: Ch 14). At the time that Balint wrote, there was a very strong theoretical inclination among psychoanalysts and their followers to disregard external contexts, so it is anachronistic to assume that such selective inattention would apply now. Nevertheless, there is still a preference in the Balint movement to subsume all discussion of wider contexts within a consideration of the doctor–patient relationship. In his guidelines for Balint groups, written on behalf of the Balint Society, Sackin has written:

> Matters of fact may need to be cleared up at points during the discussion but only those that have a bearing on the doctor/patient relationship are relevant. Discussion of general issues is also not relevant. (Sackin 1994)

Once again, it is unclear what implications this guidance regarding seminars is meant to have on the way that consultations themselves should be conducted. However, the observable effect of this kind of emphasis seems to be that many Balintian practitioners appear to prefer questions about subjective emotional experience rather than questions that contextualise that experience.

As this book has pointed out, a narrative approach places a great deal of theoretical emphasis on contexts. Drawing on contemporary practice in family therapy, narrative practitioners pay attention to how stories are influenced by family histories, culture, race, gender, class or the experience of deprivation (Nichols and Schwartz 2001). They are acutely aware of how professionals can add to their patients' distress by ignoring these contexts, or by focusing mainly on psychological issues. They also pay attention to the healthcare context itself, and how it can impair professionals and work against the interests of patients (Lindblad-Goldberg *et al.* 1998). They make direct enquiry into all these contexts, regarding this as a prerequisite for understanding the patient's utterances. There is, in other words, a much broader scope of conversation with patients. This encompasses anything that is unfamiliar or different from the interviewer's own experience. It includes the historical or social realities, as the patient perceives them, and the health service context itself.

Interpretations

Balint claimed that his work with GPs was aimed at constructing an over-arching system of psychopathology at a 'different, deeper or more comprehensive level' than the conventional medical one (Balint 1957: 38). While he was sceptical about the psychiatric approach to diagnosis, he sought to develop an alternative diagnostic system that was based on psychoanalytic interpretations and on the idea of widespread neurosis in those who consult GPs. Many of the case histories in *The Doctor, his Patient and the Illness* are formulated in terms of psychoanalytic interpretations. In a typical case, a patient's high blood pressure is put down to sexual frustration (Balint 1957: 36). The key to this aspect of his thinking perhaps appears in his central theoretical claim:

> If I am right, psychoanalysis is about to develop a new conception which may be called 'basic illness' or perhaps 'basic fault' in the biological structure of the individual, involving in varying degrees both his mind and his body. (Balint 1957: 255)

This conception, Balint suggests, should guide GPs throughout their researches and act as a framework for the way they think about their patients. Balint's thinking, like all thinking based on classical psychoanalysis, therefore centred on the assumption that there is often an underlying meaning to many of the things that doctors come across in their practice, especially the patient's symptoms, their mode of presentation and the effect on the doctor. These meanings represented some kind of truth regarding the essential nature of the problem. Discovering the nature of this truth would produce therapeutic effects, either through the patient gaining new understanding or through the generation of strong cathartic emotion, or both. Such a powerful underlying belief may have had great influence in primary care in encouraging practitioners to believe that there was always something more 'profound' or 'essential' to discover.

Balint's writing, however, is not always consistent in this respect. There is a strand of non-dogmatic, sceptical and self-critical thought that runs through much of his writing, and indeed through psychoanalytic thinking as a whole. It is a strand of thinking that regards exploration as more important than labels, and the conversation as more therapeutic than interpretations (Frosh

1997). This more flexible approach is certainly evident in some later Balint commentators, including his widow Enid Balint, and in the work of Norell, and Samuel and Elder. Salinsky demonstrates this with his claim:

> [The GP] can also be regarded as a useful person to have as a fellow traveller; able when necessary to help with the navigation or repair the engine, but mostly there to share the experience and help to reflect on it. (Salinsky 1987)

Such a claim is much closer to the narrative approach. Here, the search for meaning is seen as something which is collaborative, constantly evolving, always provisional and only truthful in so far as it produces an understanding which the patient finds helpful in some way, and for some time. Some of the leaders of the contemporary Balint movement might even see this as an accurate description of their own beliefs as much as a description of a narrative approach (Sackin 2001).

Can the two approaches be integrated?

In spite of the clear differences between the two approaches, there is clearly scope for combining elements from the two. Over many years, a number of writers and teachers have examined the possibility of using Balintian ideas together with ideas from family therapy (Hopkins 1959; Lask 1972; Glenn 1983; Botelho *et al.* 1990; Launer 1995; Johnston and Brock 2001). At the Tavistock, we have now taught many people who have a background in Balint work. A number of these report that they have started to ask circular questions, while at the same time continuing to make use of silence. Others say that they still find it useful to try and interpret the unconscious reasons for patients' problems, although they have come to see such interpretations as provisional hypotheses rather than definitive explanations. Some report that they are attempting to find a middle way between the intense empathy they were encouraged to acquire in their Balint training and the more dispassionate questioning stance that we have promoted.

Yet at the same time, the distinctions between the two approaches cannot and perhaps should not be blurred. The narrative approach that we teach makes an explicit claim to offer a more contemporary and less paternalistic way of conceptualising the consultation. We express open concern about the more abusive tendencies that have been displayed in the past by practitioners who believe they have been influenced by the Balint tradition, including examples we have seen in videos, role play or self-reported consultations. (We express even more acute concern about some of the 'received wisdom' from the related area of psychosexual medicine, where practitioners have traditionally been encouraged to seek revealing personal information about patients while carrying out vaginal examinations.)

A narrative approach also makes a claim to go beyond the areas addressed by the Balint tradition, in seeing primary care as an indivisible field. It argues that the consultation, or the doctor–patient relationship, cannot be separated from all the organisational, political, social or historical contexts that make it what it is. From a narrative point of view, direct enquiry into these contexts is not a form of emotional escapism or conversational distraction. It is an indispensable part of trying to understand what is happening in the encounter, and of making that encounter effective.

Three quotations end this chapter. They are comments from different GPs who have been members of Balint groups and have valued that experience, but have subsequently gone on to learn a narrative-based approach as well. They reflect the overall impressions of doctors who have learned both approaches, and who have offered us comments on the differences between the two.

> Balint strikes me as being mainly about training doctors to observe and identify with their patients. Any therapeutic change occurs as a result of that connection, i.e. change is spontaneous and not planned. The narrative approach is about achieving change in the patient's perceptions or beliefs about their problem through the type or focus of questions that you ask. This changes the aim of the interviewer – it is planned, conscious and led. However the final choice and responsibility lies with the patient. (Dr A)

> Balint is more interpretative, extrapolating from relationships between the patient and doctor, to the patient's other relationships. The narrative approach looks at behaviour in relationships in a variety of contexts and how each has a bearing on the other. As a GP, I see patients both alone and in larger groups with family members or friends, and this provides an ideal setting for using the narrative approach. I find great appeal in the idea that there is no ultimate universal correct answer. Remaining curious and trying to formulate hypotheses helps maintain my enthusiasm for work. It is possible to do this even working alone, even as a novice and even just doing little bits at a time. The narrative or systems approach can also be used beyond the doctor–patient relationship to look at the wider organisation of work. (Dr B)

> An essential difference for me is, for want of a better way of putting it . . . that I have come away from Balint groups with the impression that there is a right way of doing things. The lack of flexibility and alternative voices seems an important drawback. Particular strengths of the narrative approach include looking at the consultation through different lenses, for example

considering gender and cultural stories that arise in the consultation. Another useful skill is in increasing reflexivity, and considering how my own stories influence the consultation. (Dr C)

References

Balint E, Courtenay M, Elder A, Hull S and Julian D (1993) *The Doctor, the Patient and the Group: Balint revisited*. Routledge, London.

Balint E and Norell J (1973) *Six Minutes for the Patient: interactions in general practice consultations*. Tavistock, London.

Balint M (1957) *The Doctor, his Patient and the Illness*. Pitman, London.

Botelho RJ, McDaniel SH and Jones SE (1990) Using a family systems approach in a Balint style group: an innovative course for continuing medical education. *Fam Med.* **31**: 404–8.

Clyne M (1961) *Night Calls*. Tavistock, London.

Elder A (1990) Psychotherapy in general practice. In: H Maxwell (ed) *An Outline of Psychotherapy for Trainee Psychiatrists, Medical Students and Practitioners* (2e). Whurr, London.

Elder A and Samuel O (eds) (1987) *While I'm Here Doctor*. Tavistock, London.

Frosh S (1997) *For and Against Psychoanalysis*. Routledge, London.

Gill C (1979) What happened to the flash? In: P Hopkins (ed) *The Human Face of Medicine*. Pitman, London.

Glenn M (1983) Review of Balint at 25 years. *Fam Sys Med.* **1**: 75–8.

Gosling R and Turquet P (1964) The training of general practitioners. In: R Gosling, D Miller, D Woodhouse and P Turquet (eds) *The Use of Small Groups in Training*. Codicote, London.

Hopkins P (1959) Health, happiness and the family. *Br J Clin Pract.* **13**: 311–13.

Horder J (2001) The first Balint group. *Br J Gen Pract.* **51**: 1038–9.

Johnston AH and Brock CD (2001) Exploring triangulation as the foundation for family system thinking in the Balint Group process. *Fam Sys Health.* **18**: 469–78.

Lask A (1972) The role of the family and the work of the family doctor. In: P Hopkins (ed) *Patient Centred Medicine*. Pitman, London.

Launer J (1995) The doctor, the family and the system. *J Balint Soc.* **23**: 6–12.

Lindblad-Goldberg M, Dore M and Stern L (1998) *Creating Competence from Chaos: a comprehensive guide to home-based services*. Norton, New York.

Nichols MP and Schwartz RC (2001) *Family Therapy: concepts and methods* (5e). Allyn and Bacon, London.

Payne M (2000) *Narrative Therapy: an introduction for counsellors.* Sage, London.

Sackin P (2001) Personal communication.

Sackin P (1994) What is a Balint group? Statement by the Council of the Balint Society. *J Balint Soc.* **22**: 36–7.

Salinsky J (1987). Fact or fiction? In: A Elder and O Samuel (eds) *While I'm Here Doctor.* Tavistock, London.

Salinsky J (1993) *The Last Appointment*: The Book Guild, Lewes.

Salinsky J and Sackin P (2001) *How Are You Feeling, Doctor? Identifying and avoiding defensive patterns in the consultation.* Radcliffe Medical Press, Oxford.

CHAPTER 16

Towards a narrative-based model for primary care

'There is an inescapable circularity between the order of the body and the order of the text.'
Laurence Kirmayer (1992)

'We must neither disparage the body nor sacrifice the spirit.'
Abraham Joshua Heschel (1990)

This final chapter is an attempt to move towards a narrative-based model for primary care. It does so by examining one central theoretical question: how is it possible to combine a narrative-based approach with professional knowledge and expertise?

Narrative and the postmodern challenge

As the introduction to this book indicated, narrative studies come from a variety of perspectives. Some writers in this field are essentially liberal, 'modernist' ones (Kleinman 1988). They explore the way that people tell their stories. They suggest how professionals in the world of healthcare can become more attentive to those stories. However, they have little or no interest in challenging the scientific world view itself, or the way that professionals understand and use their own specialist knowledge.

By contrast, there are authors who take a much more radical and postmodern view. They understand the term narrative to cover all forms of knowledge, including science and medicine. They argue that no specialist knowledge – not even anatomy – is really 'objective', but just a set of stories that a lot of people happen to believe for the time being (Wright and Treacher 1982; Armstrong 1983, 1987). A common version of this view is that knowledge and power are synonymous, so that knowledge is the way that vested interest groups, professional or political, maintain their position and influence (Foucault 1976). Views like these quite often appear in works of medical sociology and anthropology, usually as part of a critique of the way doctors behave. They also appear in works by people in the field of mental health, including those at the more post-modern fringes of family therapy. Here is one example of such thinking:

> Scientific writing ... furnishes a no more *accurate* picture of reality than fiction. The former accounts may be embedded in scientific activity in a way that the latter are not. However, both kinds of accounts are guided by cultural conventions, historically situated, which largely determine the character of the reality they seek to depict. (Gergen and Kaye 1992)

Some people in primary care might find such views deeply unsettling. Most would probably regard them as frivolous and irrelevant, especially when set against the everyday experience of seeing people whose lives have been devastated by strokes or schizophrenia and who want the best help and the best knowledge available. These views can also seem like an affront to people who believe they are doing genuinely worthwhile work in the real world. It is therefore tempting for practitioners in primary care to dismiss postmodern ideas entirely, especially as they usually offer no guidance whatsoever as to what professionals should do when they arrive at work the next morning.

However, there are two reasons why it may be worth considering postmodern ideas like these seriously, at least as a starting point. One reason is that they can act as a helpful caution against excessive certainty. They draw attention to the way that scientific knowledge is indeed produced within specific social and political contexts (for example, the way that research is promoted by the pharmaceutical industry and by governments with particular economic agendas). They can act as a caution against the tendency of some clinicians to dismiss other bodies of knowledge, such as complementary medical systems, non-Western systems or religious beliefs. They can encourage practitioners to be more reflective and more flexible about emerging issues, such as accountability to patients and awareness of the experiences of disadvantaged people, and also in relation to working more democratically with other professions.

There is another reason for not throwing out the baby with the bath water. Scientific and medical knowledge does actually change (Kuhn 1970), sometimes radically so. We are all familiar with diseases that have vanished without trace (like neurasthenia) or been summoned into existence to explain the inexplicable (like 'irritable bowel syndrome'). We may also be aware that some conditions are regarded by different medical authorities in entirely different ways, according to their ideological perspectives, like premenstrual syndrome (Rodin 1992) or 'ME'. Most experienced practitioners can recall explaining to patients in the past how they had conditions that would now be regarded as quite different or even non-existent. The sociologist Gabbay has shown how historical descriptions of illnesses, such as asthma, can be utterly unrecognisable (Gabbay 1982). They each contain a self-referential loop of symptoms, signs, diagnosis and treatment, none of which make sense to us. The knowledge in them is no longer a story that we can understand or use.

These are good reasons for taking a postmodern view of medicine seriously. Yet there are at least two theoretical areas where a postmodernist view is highly problematical. First, how should we regard things like broken bones and death that are recognised across all histories and cultures? Second, what are people meant to do when society requires them to act in certain ways such as declaring patients to need compulsory psychiatric treatment? Although some practitioners may not be terribly bothered by these questions, at least from a theoretical point of view, it is worth grappling with them because this may help practitioners use narrative ideas more imaginatively in all the dimensions of their work.

Narrative, knowledge and action

There are two sets of ideas that offer a sensible compromise between the notion that everything, including death, is a mere story, and the notion that science is the authoritative explanation for all reality.

The first set of ideas concerns *knowledge*. It suggests that reality is neither just a story, nor entirely knowable, but somewhere in-between (Bury 1986; Speed 1991; Pocock 1995; Frosh 1995; Orange 1995; Lannaman 1998; Williams 1999). According to this view, *we can use current versions of knowledge because they are the best provisional stories we have, although we should test them against reality all the time to see how they work*. In other words, we should carry on with them as long as they seem to do the job, but reject them or adapt them when they do not. Working in this way, we should expect that some forms of story, such as death and broken bones, will generally turn out to be true, whereas others will be less so according to the context, or over time.

One advantage of this view is that it promotes a sceptical attitude to science but not a cynical one. Indeed, it resembles the scientific method itself (Popper 1959), although the kind of testing being suggested here is not of experimentation in the laboratory, but of a continual testing of stories against reality.

Another advantage of this view is that it frames all of us as participants in the creation of knowledge. It implies, for example, that in every consultation we are simultaneously applying contemporary stories about reality, testing them for their current efficacy and developing them into something different. If that is the case, then helping patients to create new narratives will not only benefit those individuals, it will also contribute towards new cultural or professional narratives. There is, in other words, a reciprocal connection between the stories our patients tell us, the new stories they go away with, the stories we tell our colleagues about them and the stories that get into the textbooks as 'medicine' (Dallos 1997).

Perhaps the greatest advantage of taking this view is that it enables professionals to get on with their everyday jobs while still being reflective. It relieves them from the anxiety that what they do is inherently oppressive, or that it only derives from self-interest. It opens up a way of working that involves both an understanding of narrative ideas and the use of expertise.

The second set of ideas concerns *action*. It justifies professional action on the grounds that *we have no choice except to act within currently accepted systems of thought*. Though we may know at an intellectual level that all systems of thought are probably unstable, we also have to realise that we cannot 'get out of the frame' of our current social circumstances. Nor can we challenge everything in the social web of meaning that sustains us and gives us our identities without putting our own professional standing and livelihood at risk. Lang and his colleagues put the point as follows:

> Human life would not be possible were it not for the fact that there are a number of episodes which we enact without self reflection, taking for granted the usefulness of the rules that hold these things together. A world of perpetual change and perpetual re-evaluation would not be liveable. The conventions of life are constructed and maintained socially, culturally and contextually. (Lang *et al.* 1990)

Such an argument suggests that, even from a sceptical viewpoint, it is fine for professionals to behave 'normally'. This does not imply that professionals have a licence to behave in a reactionary way, asserting their professional authority to act without question. Quite the reverse, it invites them to consider at every moment what opportunities there might be to function more liberally or reflectively. However, where action is clearly unavoidable within accepted professional codes of behaviour, the argument provides a justification for doctors to act decisively and without self-reproach.

Narrative and expertise: taking a dual stance

For much of their working lives, primary care professionals are called on to take an expert stance that assumes that scientific reality is an absolute truth. They talk to their patients about risk and danger, and the reality of disease and death. Their expert status authorises them to take a routine history, examine the patient's body, offer clear diagnoses, provide scientific information, give guidance on prevention and advise on treatment. It also requires them to keep up to date, run an efficient practice, follow professional and governmental guidelines, pursue good outcomes, and keep within ethical codes and the law. Many patients will wish their doctors to maintain such an expert stance for much of the time. There are also many external authorities that require them to do so.

At the same time, professionals – particularly in primary care – may often want to ask themselves questions about their expertise: '*Will I still be acting in this way in ten years time?*' or '*Are we all doing this because of fashion, or political pressure, or scarce resources?*' or '*Is this just the way we currently tell our stories about reality?*' A narrative stance encourages them to ask such questions. It allows them to let go of the pursuit of illness and treatment, and instead to ask about people's lives and emotions, in the belief that the discovery of meaning is more important than things that can be measured. It prompts them to seek out the patient's alternative explanations of reality, especially when these arise from personal experiences or so-called 'folk beliefs'. It permits them to bend the rules by prescribing antibiotics in 'questionable' cases or ordering 'unnecessary' x-rays in order to reassure people on the grounds that it is more important to help someone with their own story than to maintain one's own sense of correctness. It invites them to think about the organisational structures and social contexts in which they work, and how these might be influencing their encounters.

Both the expert stance and the narrative one have much to offer, but they may have more to offer in combination than either of them does alone. The most helpful way of approaching the work of primary care may be through maintaining a 'dual stance'. Such a stance combines the use of expertise together with intelligent questions about that expertise. *Taking a dual stance involves moving continually between a knowledge-based position and a story-making position.* It means letting narrative ideas provide a radical voice, or act as a kind of sceptical 'court jester', in relation to expertise, without being allowed to undermine it (Launer 1996).

Within primary care, there are times when narrative and expertise coincide effortlessly. This happens, for example, when a medical explanation about how the body works, or how it may go wrong, makes complete sense to the patient as a new account of their problem. It also happens when patients are entirely happy to absorb a conventional diagnosis or treatment into their own changing story. Such moments are common in everyday practice. They remind us that the 'medical story' is not just the property of one profession. It belongs collectively to our culture and our society (Lupton 1994). These moments also remind us that the practice of primary care can be about sharing knowledge and power rather than imposing it.

Conversely, there are times when expert ways of understanding what is going on are inadequate at best, and destructive at worst. These are encounters where medical accounts run the risk of making things worse: by giving biological labels to biographical experiences, by pathologising adverse life events or by codifying complexity. It is in these common circumstances that the narrative stance comes into its own, by offering not one but many perspectives, none of them exclusive.

There are also grey areas where expertise is not enough on its own. Sometimes practitioners offer a good medical story that does not really make sense to the patient. At other times the patient wants a medical story but the clinician cannot find one to fit. Or perhaps both the professional and the patient find the 'official' story partly helpful and partly not. It is at times like these that the narrative stance also comes into its own by pointing towards a different kind of story.

A better story for the patient

When the expert story does not work, or is not enough, what ideas can guide our search for good new stories for patients?

One helpful starting point is the idea of *negotiability*. This means the extent to which different accounts of reality – of the kinds explored throughout this book – might be possible in any consultation. Partly, negotiability depends on how far patients are willing to entertain different stories – for example, whether they are prepared to reframe their problem in terms of relationships, family and culture. It also depends on the ability of professionals to reflect on their own conceptual landscapes and to show genuine curiosity about different kinds of stories, perhaps ones determined by other cultures, other beliefs or other experiences. Thus, negotiability is not about persuading the patient to accept the conventional, medical view. It is about holding the problem or the story up to the light to see how many other facets there are, and how many different angles they can be viewed from.

One aid to exploring negotiability is the idea that we all possess *multiple voices* (Papadopoulos and Byng-Hall 1997). For example, a doctor may simultaneously be a senior member of the general practice profession and also gay or a widower. A nurse might be a senior manager within her team but also a refugee and a lone parent. All of us as professionals, and all of the patients whom we see, will have multiple identities: as the children of our parents, perhaps as parents of children, as workers in our professions, partners or spouses of those we live with, members of our families of origin and of our households, participants in interest groups or faith communities, and so on. We are people who treat illness but, almost inevitably, people who have suffered from illnesses ourselves in the past or are having to live with infirmities of one kind or another. We may be significantly depressed at times but function extremely well at others, or be highly independent in some contexts but helpless in others. We may wish at times to give voice to each of these identities and tell stories that derive from those identities.

Seen in this way, the task of the narrative practitioner is not to look for the sole story but to create opportunities for patients to explore a rich variety of stories, and to explore and create new ones from among them. The task may also be to focus on the exceptions rather than the rules, the chinks of light shining between the words rather than the solid blocks of darkness they appear to be. The statement '*I had a very unhappy childhood*' therefore invites questions like '*Were there particular people or places that made it bearable?*' or '*Where did you find the strength to overcome it and lead a productive life?*' The complaint '*I haven't been free of pain for years*' invites similar questions. The point of such questions is not to dismiss or belittle the patients' statements. It is to signal the rich variety of stories available for any reality, and the power we always have to choose from among these.

In looking for potential transformations of the story, there is one particular area that is often a fertile source of alternative stories. This is the area that the French historian Foucault called *subjugated discourse* (Flaskas and Humphreys 1993). According to this idea, much of our conversation, particularly when we are in a professional role, is governed by the stories that are most connected with systems of power and control, such as the professions, the social establishment, the managerial class or the state. Yet at the same time it is open to us to explore different experiences, different stories and different realities. These alternative realities include, for example, the stories people tell from the perspective of being female, or from an ethnic minority, or disabled, or socially marginalised in some way.

Practitioners who want to look for an alternative story might therefore direct their attention to the 'stories that are struggling to get out' or 'the stories of the underdog' (Thomas *et al.* 1996; Campbell 1997). The aim of doing so is to help individuals whose voices are often heard less than the dominant ones in society, and to empower them. It is also to change the stories that are more widely told within society itself, so that these may incorporate more fully the voices that had not previously been heard. The narrative role can therefore be seen as an inherently subversive one, counterbalancing the conservative role that all primary care professionals have to play in representing the 'official' stories of medicine and the state.

A better story for the professional

Very often, the story that helps the patient most is also an acceptable story for the practitioner. However, this is not always the case. If the patient is satisfied with a version of reality that leaves the practitioner deeply uncomfortable or seriously worried, that is not a good story. Professionals also seek their own narratives, and these need to correspond with wider professional and cultural stories about doing their job: narratives of doing good, avoiding harm, preventing risk and not putting themselves in any kind of danger. The narratives that professionals take away from their everyday encounters – like their patients' new stories – have to be coherent, aesthetic and useful.

Every professional sometimes see a patient who tells a narrative that seems full of ignorance and error. Sometimes the ensuing encounter does not lead to any perceptible change in this state of affairs. Clinicians are then left with exactly the same sense of distress that they tried to alleviate in the patient. In these situations, there may be no alternative to asserting the professional narrative as forcefully as is necessary. In some cases, this may even involve saying: '*As a doctor, I believe your decision is a dangerous one and I have to tell you that.*' The extreme instance of such situations is when a doctor or social worker has to invoke the Mental Health Act or take other statutory action, such as initiating a child protection referral. Although such actions are likely to be in diametric opposition to the stories that patients or parents tell about themselves, there is nothing in such actions that is inconsistent with a narrative-based approach. Quite the contrary, it affirms the importance of the contexts that determine the narrative on both sides of the conversation.

Such cases are, fortunately, rare. In most encounters, professionals do not have to impose their own narratives with such certainty or authority. A much more familiar difficulty is that of practical limitations. A satisfactory story for a patient is not a good one if it leaves the practitioner with a waiting room full of irate people who have been kept waiting, or a spouse and family who feel abandoned or with a personal sense of resentment. A narrative-based approach does not advocate self-sacrifice. It acknowledges that practitioners sometimes have to foreclose a story or take short cuts because of lack of time or for other pressing needs. A good story is one that leaves the professional's sense of job satisfaction and self-preservation intact too.

Is this always possible? The answer may be no. At the time of writing, primary care in many places is besieged. Where the pressure is great, and the support systems inadequate, it may be impossible to provide conditions that satisfy both the patients' need for meaning and the practitioners' need for personal survival. A narrative-based approach cannot by itself overcome this. It cannot wish away deprivation any more than it can wish away pain. It cannot raise taxes, distribute them equitably or pay for buildings and staff. However, there are two things it can offer in relation to extreme practical limitations. One is to invite practitioners to enquire how such a state of affairs was reached and how other colleagues in comparable situations (in other localities or in other countries) managed to fare better. The other is to point out that story telling can be used with a political purpose too. Narratives of deprivation belong not just to the consulting room but also to the professional journal, the local and national newspaper, radio and television. From there, they may bring about wider change.

Towards a narrative-based model for primary care

This book has attempted to show the many uses of narrative ideas in primary care. It has indicated how primary care can be seen as a place where vast numbers of stories intersect and in turn give rise to new stories. These stories chiefly meet in one-to-one encounters in consultations. Yet they also interact in a rich variety of other contexts, including conversations with families, discussions among colleagues, and in teaching, supervision and management. All these stories play their part in creating the reality in which primary professionals work. Primary care is, in that sense, a 'universe of stories' (Parry 1991).

Primary care lies at the crossroads between the world of stories and the world of facts. Its practitioners need to know when someone is suffering from heartache and when they are having a heart attack – and to give an appropriate response to either. Narrative offers people in this setting a liberating and sophisticated conceptual model that allows them both to use and to question their own professional expertise. However, it can never claim to be 'the sole truth'. By definition, any narrative approach must itself remain open to further questions. For the moment, it can perhaps suggest a form of words to describe our working reality – but that form of words will in time lose its meaning and that reality too will change. Narrative may seem an idea that is right for now but, like all ideas, it is provisional. If narrative is to remain narrative, the phrase 'towards a theory . . . ' can never lose the word 'towards'.

Some people who have read this book may choose to take on a narrative-based approach wholeheartedly, either by deciding to learn more about it formally on a course or by exploring it in their own workplaces. Some readers may take on a few ideas and incorporate these with ideas from other approaches into their own personal synthesis. Perhaps a few will develop a narrative approach in ways that take it very far from anything described here. Readers will all have made their own stories out of the foregoing pages, and these stories will carry on after they have closed the book.

References

Armstrong D (1983) *Political Anatomy of the Body*. Cambridge University Press, Cambridge.

Armstrong D (1987) Bodies of knowledge: Foucault and the problem of human anatomy. In: D Scambler (ed) *Sociological Theory and Medical Sociology*. Tavistock, London.

Bury M (1986) Social constructionism and the development of medical sociology. *Soc Health Illn.* **8**: 135–69.

Campbell D (1997) The other side of the story: the clients' experience of therapy. In: R Papadopoulos and J Byng-Hall (eds) *Multiple Voices: narrative in systemic family psychotherapy.* Duckworth, London.

Dallos R (1997) *Interacting Stories: narratives, family beliefs and therapy.* Karnac, London.

Flaskas C and Humphreys C (1993) Theorising about power: intersecting the ideas of Foucault with the 'problem' of power in family therapy. *Fam Proc.* **32**: 35–47.

Foucault M (1976) *The Birth of the Clinic.* Tavistock, London.

Frosh S (1995) Post-modernism versus psychotherapy. *J Fam Ther.* **17**: 175–90.

Gabbay J (1982) Asthma attacked? Tactics for the reconstruction of a disease concept. In: T Wright and A Treacher (eds) *The Problem of Medical Knowledge: examining the social construction of medicine.* Edinburgh University Press, Edinburgh.

Gergen K and Kaye J (1992) Beyond narrative in the negotiation of therapeutic meaning. In: S McNamee and K Gergen (eds) *Therapy as Social Construction.* Sage, London.

Heschel AJ (1990) *Quest for God: studies in prayer and symbolism.* Crossroad, New York.

Kirmayer L (1992) The body's insistence on meaning: metaphor as presentation and representation in illness experience. *Med Anth Q.* **6**: 323–46.

Kleinman A (1988) *The Illness Narratives: suffering, healing and the human condition.* Basic Books, New York.

Kuhn T (1970) *The Structure of Scientific Revolutions.* University of Chicago, Chicago.

Lang WP, Little M and Cronen V (1990) The systemic professional: domains of action and the question of neutrality. *Hum Sys.* **1**: 39–55.

Lannaman NJ (1998) Social construction and materiality: the limits of indeterminacy in therapeutic settings. *Fam Proc.* **37**: 393–413.

Launer J (1996) 'You're the doctor, Doctor!': is social constructionism a helpful stance in general practice consultations? *J Fam Ther.* **18**: 255–67.

Lupton D (1994) *Medicine as Culture: illness, disease and the body in Western societies.* Sage, London.

Orange D (1995) *Emotional Understanding: studies in psychoanalytic epistemology.* Guilford, New York.

Papadopoulos R and Byng-Hall J (eds) (1997) *Multiple Voices: narrative in systemic family psychotherapy.* Duckworth, London.

Parry A (1991) A universe of stories. *Fam Proc.* **30**: 37–54.

Pocock D (1995) Searching for a better story: harnessing modern and post-modern positions in family therapy. *J Fam Ther.* **17**: 149–73.

Popper K (1959) *The Logic of Scientific Discovery.* Hutchinson, London.

Rodin M (1992) The social construction of premenstrual syndrome. *Soc Sci Med.* **35**: 49–56.

Speed B (1991) Reality exists OK? An argument against constructivism and social construc-
    tionism. *J Fam Ther.* **13**: 395–409.

Thomas P, Romme M and Hamelijnck J (1996) Psychiatry and the politics of the underclass.
    Br J Psychiatry. **169**: 401–4.

Williams SJ (1999) Is anybody there? Critical realism, chronic illness and the disability
    debate. *Soc Health Illn.* **21**: 797–819.

Wright P and Treacher A (1982) *The Problem of Medical Knowledge.* Edinburgh University
    Press, Edinburgh.

Appendix: the initial research

This appendix describes the consultation research that gave us the idea for a primary care training. The research arose from a wish to explore the relevance of contemporary ideas from family therapy to primary care. It was informed by the current family therapy literature and, in particular, by ideas in some of the sources quoted in this book. Although the ideas presented in this book have developed considerably in the years since the original research was done, readers may find it helpful to know more about how the seeds of these ideas were first sown.

The research was based on the GP consultation, and it addressed one simple question: *if you look at consultations as encounters where meaning is continuously being created, what do you see?*

The method used in the research was 'grounded theory': this means looking closely at what went on in consultations, in order to generate new theoretical ideas (Glaser and Strauss 1967; Henwood and Pidgeon 1992). This is not the only way of carrying out narrative research (Strauss and Corbin 1990; Guba and Lincoln 1994). Other approaches include discourse analysis (Elwyn and Gwyn 1998) and performative approaches (Langellier 1989). However, grounded theory is a particularly useful approach for developing theory in areas where this is lacking. The method was used because it seemed that primary care lacked a contemporary theoretical framework, compared with the relatively clear one that had emerged for family therapy.

The material used was video and audiotapes of consultations, and their transcripts. These were examined repeatedly in the light of the research question, trying to identify which common themes emerged. In summary, these were the findings.

- Consultations can be seen as attempts to create an agreed new story that satisfies the beliefs and understanding of both the doctor and the patient.
- A number of important themes or contexts within the consultation need to be negotiated in order to develop a new story. These include such things as time, task, personal distance, action, explanations and suffering.
- Many external contexts also influence how the story evolves. For the patient, these include family, culture and previous encounters with healthcare. For the professional, they include workload, evidence and money.

- Consultations may or may not produce a satisfactory new story. When they do not, it may be because narrative threads have not been followed through. It may also be because important contexts of one kind or another have not been openly stated nor adequately discussed.

What follows is an expansion of these ideas. First there is a description of the setting, then the research findings are illustrated with excerpts from consultations and with descriptions of two whole consultations. Finally, there is a discussion of the findings and their implications.

How do clinics affect narratives?

No conversation is intelligible without knowing how it is affected by its immediate contexts – the context of the setting and the context of the relationships within the setting. The practice where the research took place was in a health centre, built in the 1970s. Most of the patients were from social classes III, IV and V. About a third of the practice's patients were of non-British ethnic origin. At the time of the research, the practice was a five-partner practice, entirely within the NHS. There was a team of employed and 'attached' professionals, including GP registrars and a nurse practitioner, together with practice nurses, health visitors, a community midwife, district nurses and a specialist nurse for the terminally ill. The practice shared the building with other agencies, including school nurses, chiropodists and community paediatricians.

How might such a setting influence the conversations taking place and the kind of stories generated there? Within the context of British general practice, large group practices in urban health centres represent a particular subculture. Many GPs who work in such settings choose to do so because of a particular set of values, including commitment to a public health service and a belief in teamwork. Some patients may register because they believe that a large group practice in a publicly owned building provides a better service, and they might think it a privilege to belong to it – although others might see it as an impersonal, even hostile public institution, and the people who work there as professional failures.

Like every practice, this one had a particular practice style. Each patient was registered with a named doctor, with the declared purpose of encouraging personal continuity of care. Doctors and nurses, who all dressed informally, came into the waiting room to summon patients personally. Doctors used separate examining rooms attached to the consulting rooms and always used chaperones when male doctors carried out physical examinations on women. Such behaviour was intended to represent characteristic beliefs and values concerning social equality and equity. It was, of course, open to patients to construe this behaviour in many different ways. They might have seen it in a positive light or as evidence of aberrance. However these factors might operate, they would all have an impact on the encounters between doctors and patients, the conversations that took place and the stories that it was possible to create.

How do surgery rules affect narratives?

Institutions like health centres have effects on the conversations that take place within them, but so does the nature of the surgeries themselves. As well as looking at the practice setting in our research, the research also looked at how surgeries were composed. We noticed, for example, that different doctors saw varying numbers of unbooked patients during their sessions. Officially, the practice restricted unbooked attendances to cases 'in need of urgent medical attention'. However, patients varied in their perceptions of urgent need and in their assertiveness when requesting attention. GPs differed in their willingness to have their scheduled work disrupted and in their readiness to resist pressing demands (and risk the consequent moral, disciplinary and medicolegal penalties).

Even more noticeable were the rules – spoken and unspoken – regarding consultation length. In theory, doctors saw patients who were booked at seven-and-a-half-minute intervals (technically patients were asked to come at 9.00, 9.05, 9.15, etc., to give an average length of seven-and-a-half minutes.) Yet there was a large difference between average consultation times and in how much doctors would extend the time. This pointed towards significant ways in which the nature of consultations may be determined. For example, short consultations have the potential to be highly compressed and efficient, and they allow the doctor to remain punctual. However, they obviously run the risk of imposing stories that are hasty, superficial and stereotyped. Long consultations have the opposite potential: unpunctuality on the one hand, but the chance of developing more measured and reflective narratives.

The surgeries differed in their 'dramatis personae', highlighting some of the ways in which surgery lists may reflect the preferences of practices, doctors and patients. There were differences in gender, age, ethnicity and in the number of patients accompanied by parents or spouses. There were also differences in the nature of the problems brought to the doctors. Only a few consultations could be described as single episodes, concerning self-limiting conditions and not deriving from a previous contact nor leading to another one being planned. All the others were part of a continuing involvement with doctors, often one that spanned many years and possibly three or four family generations. Few consultations ended in a specialist referral. This suggested that there was a particular practice style: one that privileged continuing medical management over crisis intervention and where primary care was seen as the preferred locus for the vast majority of medical conversations.

Finally, in every surgery there were non-attendances. These may have had a variety of meanings, including clerical errors, simple forgetfulness and expressions of displeasure with the doctor. Because appointments were so short, patients might not have thought it necessary to make cancellations. A corollary of this is that attenders may not have believed that their presence or punctuality was valued. One of the interesting features of a service that is free at the point of delivery is that GPs cannot apply sanctions to non-attenders (even in repeated instances) short of the drastic one of removing them from the list. This limitation may affect rates of attendance, but may also have had its own influence on those who did choose to keep their appointment. Among the many and varied factors that go to make up a context in primary care, none can fail to have an effect on the conversations that take place there and on the conversations that can or cannot take place. Alter any one aspect of the context, and the stories will change.

Narrative in the consultation: six contexts in search of a story

This section describes what went on in the consultations themselves. Through a close examination of passages from the transcripts, it shows how patients and doctors negotiate certain important themes or contexts in consultations in order to construct an agreed new story.

When patients and doctors take up the initial narrative – often puzzling or incomplete – that the patient has brought in, they work on it together in an attempt to produce something different and more satisfactory. As they do so, it seems that they need to negotiate a few essential contexts in order to move forward. Some of these contexts provide an agreed framework for a new narrative to develop (for example, 'how much time do we have?'). Others are crucial to the content of the narrative itself ('I want to tell you how I am feeling'). From examining the consultations that were recorded, six contexts emerged as particularly important. They were:

- time
- task
- personal distance
- action
- explanation
- suffering.

These were clearly not the only ones that might be identified, and further examination (or examination of other consultations) might have highlighted a wide range of further contexts. However, the research concentrated on an analysis of these six contexts in particular. They can be seen as a set of lenses for examining the material, each of which may show up a different kind of graining or detail.

Time: 'How long have we got?'

In a GP surgery, consultations are extremely short and often of indefinite length. Patients may not know the intended length of their appointments. Furthermore, many practices do not make this length explicit when patients book or when they arrive. Consultations commonly overrun, so that patients later in the surgery may have long waiting times. There is often pressure from the doctor to hasten consultations and pressure from patients to extend them. In addition, GPs and their patients may not have clear contracts regarding review appointments: for example, how often they should be, over how long a period or whether they are needed at all. Such arrangements are traditionally made from consultation to consultation.

It is therefore not surprising to find that many exchanges between patients and doctors feature implicit or explicit attempts to address the context of time, in order to set some clear boundaries for the narrative. Here, for example, a mother has just brought her child along to take up an appointment she had originally booked for herself. Once the doctor has seen the child, this exchange takes place.

Patient: This appointment was originally for me.
Doctor: Um.
Patient: To have my coil removed. Can I make that in a morning surgery?
Doctor: Yes, it doesn't have to be morning or evening.
Patient: I'm going to go on the 'mini-pill'. Would it be possible to have a prescription?
Doctor: In fact, you're asking for the 'mini-pill' before you have the coil out, right?
Patient: I was wondering, yeah. I don't know how long your appointments are.

In consultations like these, there are attempts by patients to establish the ground rules concerning time. Often, the doctors' responses can be quite oblique. It is often unclear who has 'won' in the allocation of time and how it should be used. The new narrative is often created in the end only by discussing the content of problems.

The next patient asks for her child to be seen too. The doctor tries to combine comments about time with education about how to judge whether a consultation is really necessary.

Patient: I brought Jessica along with me because . . . can you listen to her chest please?

Doctor: Right, Jessica, let's have a listen. She certainly looks very well. Chest is clear.

Patient: Oh that's OK then. So it's just in her throat then.

Doctor: Yes, yes. If she's well and not vomiting it's highly unlikely to be a significant problem on her chest.

Patient: That's all right then.

Doctor: No, I'm just thinking in future if you're trying to work out whether . . .

Patient: Yes, but I thought as I was coming I'd ask you.

Doctor: OK then.

Task: 'The kind of service I want you to perform'

Typically in consultations, the patient presents an initial story of a complaint that seems to imply the context: 'I want you to do something for me'. The doctor then develops an assumption about what this task is: diagnosis, reassurance, witnessing, facilitating hospital appointments and so on. However, as they try to develop the story, it is striking how often both the doctor and the patient only hint at these tasks rather than agreeing to define them overtly.

Patient: These tablets I'm taking for diabetes . . . you asked me if I had any side effects. Would they make you feel tired?

Doctor: Is that what you're noticing?

Patient: Well, I am noticing. I sort of feel tired. Whether it's me, I don't know, but when I get to bed . . . I'm very short-tempered. I noticed that with my grandson the other day because I had him all day.

In the next few minutes of this particular consultation, the doctor makes a number of attempts to judge whether the patient's feelings are a 'side effect', but the patient has clearly forgotten this was her reason for mentioning them. Fairly soon, the doctor settles on the task of witnessing the patient's feelings of tiredness and irritability. The initial 'formal' task of taking a blood test reviewing medication is completed very quickly about 15 minutes later.

Here is another example of the way that the theme of the task is addressed.

Patient: I'm not too bad really, actually. I've come back about the results
           of those blood tests.
Doctor: Um.
Patient: And also I went to have a scan, and it was all clear. There's noth-
           ing there at all.
Doctor: [Looks at notes] The blood tests first of all.

Unilaterally, the doctor has selected the first topic – the blood test – as the
initial task and goes on to explain that the blood test was negative. However,
as the consultation progresses, it becomes clear that the patient is quite uncon-
cerned about this, so the doctor moves to the second topic – the normal scan
result:

Doctor: Right, and then the other thing is the pain in your tummy. Well,
           that's good news.
Patient: Well yes, but what was causing it?

These extracts show that the complaint is often understood as some kind of
request to select a task, but this may not be clarified. Usually, though not
always, the doctor chooses what the main task is and this becomes the main or
even the sole focus of the new narrative.

Personal distance: 'Who are we to each other?'

In many ways, the GP consultation resembles a social situation. GPs may know
several generations of the same family over many years, and in Britain they
may often visit their homes. Patients are likely to know (and to enquire) about
the doctor's home life, holidays and hobbies. Here are two extracts which show
some rather tentative discussion about what may and may not be shared.

Patient: Did you have a nice Easter?
Doctor: Very nice, thank you.
Patient: Did you go home?
Doctor: Did I go home? I spent it with my family.
Patient: No, I mean to your home.
Doctor: Where do you imagine my home is?
Patient: Jerusalem?
Doctor: That's not my home – I have relations there.
Patient: I know you've been there.

Doctor: I've been there and I have relations there but here is very much
          my home. Here is where I was born and where I've always lived.
Patient: Oh really?
Doctor: Yes.

Patient: [Noticing the doctor's new wedding ring]: What's that?
Doctor: Have a guess.
Patient: Ooh. God bless you. Lovely. Wonderful.
Doctor: [Laughs] It's a secret. No, not really a secret.
Patient: Not any more. [Laughs]
Doctor: Take care. Bye.
Patient: Bye.

The purpose of these exchanges appears to be to set a personal context for the
evolving story. The patient and doctor subtly (or not so subtly) try to influence
each other to define the nature of the relationship.

Action: 'What I want you to do'

In many GP consultations, patients want doctors to do particular things. How
is action integrated into the story? Here are some more excerpts that demonstrate this.

Doctor: There's something I need, which is to take a blood specimen. Did
          I warn you of that?
Patient: No.
Doctor: Well, I've been checking your notes.
Patient: I know it's some time.
Doctor: It is some time.

Here, 'checking the notes' presumably refers to the doctor's duty to monitor disease and the effects of medication. None of this is spelled out, however.
    In this next consultation, action is hinted at, but never happens.

Patient: I mean, the last really bad attack was before I saw you, and you
          gave me those antibiotics.
Doctor: Yes.
Patient: And I think they did make a big difference . . .
Doctor: Right. So you're not getting pain now?
Patient: No, not like I was. I do feel sick some of the time, most of the time.
Doctor: Do antacids help?
Patient: No, they didn't really . . .

The doctor then asks some more diagnostic questions, resulting in the following exchange.

Doctor: Had anything seemed to improve it?
Patient: I do think the antibiotics made a very big difference.
Doctor: Right.
Patient: I think they made a difference.
Doctor: Right, right.

There is a clear assertion here from the patient that antibiotics helped previously, but this does not elicit an offer from the doctor, nor does the patient actually request them. Both these consultations, as well as others, indicate that action is more likely than the other themes of the consultation to be taken according to the professional, biomedical view of the world rather than the wider sociocultural one. However, it does seem possible to seek consent for this, so that action or inaction is spelt out and integrated into the final story, as the next excerpt shows.

Doctor: I don't think we need to make any sort of decision today, do you? This meeting has really been about meeting each other for the first time and establishing basic facts. Is that OK?
Patient: That's fine.

Explanation: 'What is causing this?'

Many consultations, wholly or in part, appear to be about the search for explanatory narratives concerning the patient's symptoms or subjective experiences. The following are some examples.

Patient: It's just a generalised virus?
Doctor: It seems so. He does have a slightly red throat and his glands are up. His tummy's nice and soft.
Patient: The tummy ache's nothing? It just comes with the temperature, does it?
Doctor: It just comes with the temperature.
Patient: So that's nothing to worry about. He feels giddy.
Doctor: That will go with the temperature.

Doctor: What do you think the biggest factor is in all this?
Patient: Well, I've just finished sorting out Nick's estate.

Patient: Well, I'd run out of water tablets. So would it be that? The fluid is stretching it, isn't it?

Doctor: [Examines patient] I think this is likely to be a combination of things. I think running out of water tablets may well be a factor, but I also think arthritis may be contributing to this as well.

Patient: It's such an unknown thing, ME. It's very frightening when you first get it. It frightened the life out of me. You think you're going to go down with something awful, you know. You get all sorts of things really, headaches and all kinds of aches and pains, things like that, you know ... I can't walk around shopping now for more than half an hour, but I think that's quite good even doing that, really.

In all these cases, and in many others, there is an oscillation in the developing narrative between the patient's own contributions to the developing story (or lack of them) and the doctor's. The aim of the discussion in every case appears to be to achieve a story that involves normalisation or agreement between medical and lay frameworks. This purpose often takes precedence over strictly scientific accuracy. The final explanatory narrative may have only a partial connection with biomedical science. Mostly, it seems to lie somewhere between a loose biomedical hypothesis and an essentially linguistic agreement between doctor and patient.

Suffering: 'How am I going to feel?'

Patients come to doctors with pain, anxiety, discomfort or dysphoria. The implicit purpose of every consultation is to lessen or abolish these sensations. How does the theme of suffering evolve in the course of the consultation? Here are two excerpts from consultations which suggest ways in which this happens.

Patient: I'm a bit worried about my sister actually. She's got to go in and have another camera put down her throat ... [she talks for several minutes about this] .... But I just don't know what they are going to find, you know, and I suppose this is playing on my mind. But other than that ... I'm OK really.

Patient: I mean, I think it's stress. That's what my husband says it is.

Doctor: Stress of all the children?

Patient: Yes, and just ... I think it's sort of coping with them.

Doctor: Um, um.

Patient: That's what I think it is. Lack of sleep and so on ...

Doctor: Do you get a break at all?
Patient: From the little ones? No. I mean apart from going to work. No.
Doctor: No relaxing break? Just going to work?
Patient: [Laughs] And even now, that . . . they've all been ill. Bugs, two of them. And my husband's got chicken pox. [Child coughs.]

What appears to be happening here is that there is an unstated agreement between doctor and patient that talking during a consultation is helpful. As talking proceeds, suffering itself is redefined in new language so that it is experienced as lessening. There are even occasions when the conversation is itself defined as therapeutic.

Patient: I'm really browned off. When I was in the hospital they took me off all my old pills . . .

[Some minutes pass while the doctor carefully explains the purpose of each new pill and the patient expresses her appreciation of this]

Patient: Actually, I was really impressed by the doctors in the hospital. I was quite pleased with the treatment I got there. It's only that I felt so disoriented.

Patient: I only wanted to come and talk to you. I feel it's nice to come and see you and discuss it for five minutes. Thanks ever so much then. I'll see you some time or the other. You keep well, as well!
Doctor: Thanks.

New stories that don't work, new stories that do

What distinguishes the production of a good new story from the production of a less satisfactory one? An analysis of two typical consultations offers some clues.

Consultation 1

The first consultation is between a male doctor and a young woman of Mauritian origin who speaks with a strong French accent but is otherwise fairly fluent in English. It is evidently her first meeting with the doctor. After a brief introduction, the doctor says, '*You've come for a smear then*', which the woman confirms. The doctor then embarks on a series of factual questions. Has the patient had a smear before, and when? Was her previous smear her first? When was her last period and was it normal? Have there been any problems with irregular bleeding? Is she using contraception of any kind? After this, the video camera is switched off as the two leave the room for a cubicle where a chaperone joins them and the cervical smear is carried out.

On their return, the doctor gives an explanation about smears: they are designed not to pick up cancer but pre-cancerous changes in the cells, although they do pick up cancer as well. At this point the patient enquires about whether they can detect *feebroids*. The doctor interprets this as fibroids, and explains that the smear cannot detect these, although her internal examination would have done so if they had been present.

The next part of the consultation is evidently a muddle. The patient is not sure that the doctor has understood *feebroids* and says she is worried about them because she once had a *kist* while she was pregnant. She is unsure what a *kist* is in English, and rejects the word 'cyst' when the doctor suggests it, although her description of it and her hand gestures strongly imply that this is exactly what it was. The doctor enquires what happened to this *kist* (whatever it might have been) and establishes that it was removed in the United States and was not cancerous. The doctor also enquires if the American doctors said it would cause any trouble in the future. The patient says she was told it would not. The doctor then reverts to a series of enquiries about other problems and previous pregnancies (and elicits the information that the patient has had two children and two abortions). The doctor closes the consultation with the words: '*OK. That's it then*'.

Commentary. In the context of modern general practice, this is a brisk, efficient and logical consultation. The patient has booked for a standard preventive screening measure. The doctor elicits the relevant menstrual history beforehand, explains the rationale for the procedure and later elicits a fairly full gynaecological history. Both doctor and patient, it appears, share certain cultural beliefs: in preventive medicine, in cervical smears as a legitimate part of this and in general practice as an appropriate setting for these to be performed.

At a narrative level, however, the consultation is unsatisfactory. The complicated muddle about *feebroids* and the *kist* is never resolved into a story that both doctor and patient can understand and agree. There is also no way of knowing how important it might be for the patient to find a way of giving more coherence to her narrative about her body, although there are a number of indications that she wants to try and do so. The doctor accepts the reported diagnosis of her unknown American colleague that the *kist* was benign, although it is unclear if the patient herself has fully understood or accepted that. What is certainly clear is that the doctor's chosen task has taken priority over the demands of the narrative.

Within the wider context, there are a number of possible influences that may have led to this. Cervical smears have to be performed for purely business reasons in general practice, and GPs can be financially penalised for failing to reach percentage targets in their female populations. Connected with this fact is a bureaucratic context: the doctor has to fill in a laboratory form and (at the time this research was done) an additional claim form. The doctor clearly asks some questions for this reason as much as for purely medical ones. Quite aside from the bureaucratic context, the doctor is likely to see taking smears as a correct, empowering action for the patient. It may be that the educational explanation about smears has this as its motive. Yet taken together, the need for an agreed and coherent narrative has somehow got lost.

Looked at in terms of narrative development, we can see that there are two apparent difficulties here. The first is that the doctor and patient do not establish an agreement over the meaning of certain words. (The problem in this instance is particularly highlighted by the fact that they do not speak the same first language, but may not arise solely for that reason.) The second difficulty is that the doctor chooses to remain within a professional set of contexts – including good preventive medicine and profitability. The doctor does not explore the possibility of framing the consultation in terms of the patient's contexts, for example anxiety about serious illness or just uncertainty about how she should understand what is going on within her body.

Consultation 2

This consultation shows a 13-year-old boy of African origin who has come with his mother to tell the doctor he has a swelling under his right nipple. The doctor, a woman, asks a series of questions: What made him notice it? Was it on one side or both? Does he know anybody else who has this? What does he think caused it? What goes through his mind about it?

The boy's mother then volunteers that he has another swelling on his wrist, possibly the result of a fall. The doctor asks if she thinks the two are connected and she says yes – maybe the nipple swelling was also from a fall, as he goes roller blading. The doctor examines the child and then gives two diagnoses, saying the two lumps are both harmless, and not connected. One is a ganglion. The other is gynaecomastia, which the doctor explains as a typical swelling of the fat underneath the nipple in pubertal boys. Neither need treatment.

The doctor asks if they have any questions and he says no, but his mother adds that she has noticed other 'signs of adolescence'. The GP asks what, and she says that his voice is deepening. At the same time, the boy says *spots*, and the mother then adds: '*He's having sex education too . . . that's why he got worried.*' The doctor repeats the reassurance and the mother says: '*It's always best to come for a check-up.*' Body language on the video suggests that mother and son are relieved.

Commentary. This consultation starts with the presentation of a clearly problematical story: two lumps that are possibly abnormal and dangerous. It ends with a better one: both lumps are harmless, and indeed one of them can be connoted as a sign of healthy life cycle development. It is possible that the boy may be offering another problematical story towards the end of the consultation when he says 'spots', and the doctor chooses, for whatever reason, not to explore this. It is also arguable that the family might have benefited if the doctor had tried to unpack what the mother wished to imply by her mention of sex education. Given these reservations, however, it is clear that the original story has been successfully transformed into a different narrative that appears to satisfy both mother and son.

Although there is no discussion about the purpose of the consultation, it seems as if there is implicit clarity about this. The family are visiting the doctor as a diagnostic expert who will reassure or advise them. The GP agrees to take this role. Although she takes an exploratory role in finding out about their own beliefs, she subsumes this within the role of expert when she delivers a diagnosis, explanation and advice.

One noticeable feature of this consultation is that the development of the new narrative is a joint enterprise between the doctor and the family. Each utterance by any of the participants appears to follow closely from the previous one and not to be determined by extraneous thoughts or unchecked assumptions. For example, the doctor asks enough questions to determine the nature of the story that needs alteration. Once she has offered her own new story in terms of diagnosis and reassurance, she invites further comment on it. This gives the family an opportunity to reclaim the refashioned narrative as their own. The mother takes this up and develops it into a story of normal male growth. The consultation therefore seems free of muddle for two reasons. One is that there is an unspoken agreement on the task and this sets a framework for joint working on the story. The other is that the doctor and the family follow and develop each other's narrative threads.

Bringing forth new meaning: new stories for old

Looking at consultations in terms of narrative, a number of things become clear. One is that consultations do indeed create new stories. They do so at astonishing speed. Although the brevity of the average GP consultation exerts a negative pressure on the process of story making (*'What can one possibly create in ten minutes?'*) it can also exert a positive pressure (*'We have only ten minutes, so what do we have to focus on?'*). Story making in the consultation can also incorporate all sorts of other elements such as expertise, action and education.

Language is crucial in the creation of new stories. Patients offer enormous numbers of words, all of which are potential cues. Clearly, the doctor cannot respond to every single one. But equally clearly, the doctor can ignore so many that the development of the plot is severely hampered or brought to a halt. Where communication goes wrong, it often seems to be because the doctor is following not the patient's own words, but thoughts inside his or her own head. These may have little or no connection to the words themselves, and often there is no explanation of what the thoughts are. This leads to sudden leaps in the conversation and an impediment to the progress of the new story.

Communication especially seems to go wrong when the doctor ignores words that refer to one of the main contexts that need to be agreed, such as: what is the task at hand, how much time do we have to address it and what do you want me to do?

As well as the contexts within the consultation, there are the wider contexts that give sense to the words. There is the practice setting itself, with its rules about appointment times and unbooked patients. There are the culture, class, ethnicity, age and gender of doctor and patient, and whether they are the same or (as is usually the case) in some respect different. There is all the patient's previous experience of healthcare, and all the conversations that have taken place with family and friends about the problem. There is the pressure of time, the need for the doctor to follow professional codes of evidence and of ethics, and the wish to be seen as humane and competent, as well as to make money and to stay on the right side of the law. Even this list is a mere fraction of the contexts that give meaning to the evolving story.

It is clearly impossible for the doctor to explore every one of these, just as it is impossible to follow every nuance of language. Some of the contexts will be so obvious that there is no need to discuss them (for example: '*We are in a surgery, and we have met many times before*'). There are some other contexts that the doctor may pick up intuitively without any need to enquire (for example: '*You want me to be more of a listener than an adviser today*'). In addition, there are contexts that are entirely irrelevant to the narrative (for example: '*It is July and the sun is shining*'). However, the crucial point seems to be that there will *always* be some contexts that need proper exploration if there is to be any chance of a satisfactory new story emerging. These especially seem to include people's past experience of healthcare, their family environment, and their beliefs and expectations. There are also the two core questions of every primary care encounter: '*Why me?*' (as opposed to asking someone else for help) and '*Why now?*'

Central to the creation of a new story is how the doctor makes a choice of which words and contexts to pursue. He or she may choose trivial and marginal ones, or hit a series of bullseyes. Feedback from the patient often seems to indicate which of these has occurred. An injudicious choice may call forth puzzlement, irritation or bored politeness. The doctor has, for that moment at least, lost the plot. An accurate and productive choice will meet with enthusiasm and warmth. The doctor has picked up the right language and can now develop the story further.

References

Elwyn G and Gwyn R (1998) Stories we hear and stories we tell . . . Analysing talk in clinical practice. In: T Greenhalgh and B Hurwitz (eds) *Narrative Based Medicine: dialogue and discourse in clinical practice.* BMJ Books, London.

Glaser B and Strauss A (1967) *The Discovery of Grounded Theory: strategies for qualitative research.* Aldine, New York.

Guba E and Lincoln Y (1994) Competing paradigms in qualitative research. In: NK Denzin and Y Lincoln (eds) *Handbook of Qualitative Research.* Sage, London.

Henwood K and Pidgeon N (1992) Qualitative research and psychological theorizing. *Br J Psychol.* **83**: 97–111.

Langellier K (1989) Personal narratives: perspectives on theory and research. *Text Perform Q.* **9**: 243–76.

Strauss A and Corbin J (1990) *Basics of Qualitative Research.* Sage, Newbury Park, CA.

Index